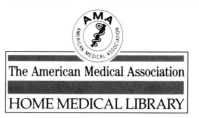

The American Medical Association

HOME MEDICAL LIBRARY

MONITORING YOUR HEALTH

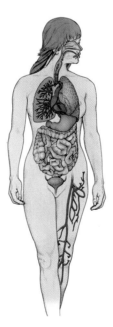

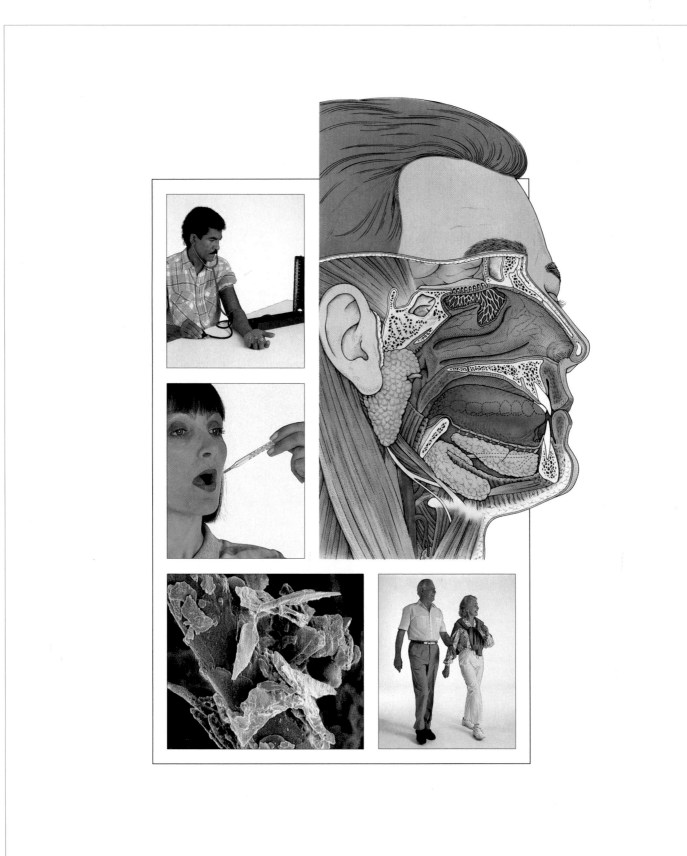

THE AMERICAN
MEDICAL ASSOCIATION

MONITORING
YOUR HEALTH

Medical Editor
CHARLES B. CLAYMAN, MD

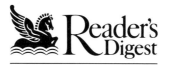

THE READER'S DIGEST ASSOCIATION, INC.
Pleasantville, New York/Montreal

Library of Congress Cataloging in Publication Data

Monitoring your health/medical editor, Charles B. Clayman.
     p.   cm. — (The American Medical Association home medical library)
    At head of title: The American Medical Association.
    Includes index.
    ISBN 0-89577-383-X
    1. Health. 2. Medicine, Preventive. I. Clayman, Charles B.
  II. American Medical Association. III. Series.
RA776.M743   1991
613 — dc20

                                               90-19348

FOREWORD

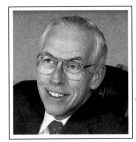

A comprehensive definition of health goes far beyond absence of disease or infirmity. Today we can consider good health to be a state of physical, mental, and social well-being. Just as we have learned a great deal about disease and injury and how to treat them, we have also learned much about good health.

One of the most significant concepts to emerge from medical studies over the last several decades is the importance of our personal health practices. We now know that good health is in part a series of decisions about how we take care of our bodies over the course of a lifetime. Our understanding of the benefits of such factors as a healthy diet, regular exercise, and stress management puts good health within the reach of more people than ever before. Many of the diseases that afflict American adults can be successfully prevented or treated by modifying aspects of our life-style. Taking these positive steps toward good health can significantly improve our physical condition and, just as importantly, put us more nearly in control of our own well-being.

Of course, not all illnesses or disabilities are preventable. Some diseases may run in your family or have less obvious causes than your life-style. Because so many diseases are treatable today, it makes good sense to learn to recognize signs and symptoms of common conditions. Prompt testing can often detect disease at an early, treatable stage.

It is easy to avoid thinking about disease or death when you are enjoying good health. However, every visit to your doctor, for a health checkup or for treatment of an illness, is an opportunity for you and your doctor to discuss how you can improve your overall health and prevent disease or infirmity.

In the chapters of this book, we at the American Medical Association offer suggestions to help you become an active, lifetime participant in your own health care.

James S. Todd, MD

JAMES S. TODD, MD
Executive Vice President
American Medical Association

CONTENTS

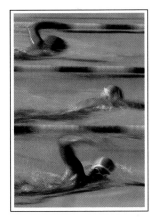

CHAPTER ONE

A LIFETIME OF GOOD HEALTH

THE HEALTH REVOLUTION in developed countries over the last 100 years has changed our perceptions of a normal life span. Up until this century, people could expect to live between 40 and 50 years. However, most people born today in developed countries can expect to live beyond 70 years of age.

No matter where or how we live, aging is a natural process. When growth is complete at the end of childhood, the brain has about 10 billion nerve cells and the kidneys have about 2 million filter units (nephrons). These numbers are far more than we need, which is why a young adult can lose a kidney or even most of a lung with little or no serious effect. However, over the course of a lifetime, the number of brain cells and nephrons declines, and the lungs grow stiffer and less able to exchange gases. Some scientists believe that the life span of our organs and tissues is genetically determined and programmed into the function of our cells. We still are not certain why physical decline occurs with age but, eventually, all the spare capacity of our vital organs is gone. Even a minor illness may be fatal. By the time most people are 85 to 90 years old, one or more organ systems usually have lost much of their functional capacity (from disease or other causes), and death results. In many areas of the world, an increasing number of men and women are approaching this advanced age.

The next goal, according to gerontologists (people who study aging), should be for more people to stay healthy until they reach their natural life expectancy. Many people who reach old age today are in poor health. If we can learn to better preserve quality of life as well as maintain vital organs throughout a lifetime, people need not be apprehensive about the prospect of advanced age.

So what is the key to staying healthier longer? Some factors are unalterable, such as the genes we inherit from our parents and some aspects of our environment. However, we can influence many of the characteristics of aging. For example, aging of the skin is accelerated by exposure to sunlight and by tobacco smoking. Flexibility of our joints can be prolonged by moderate exercise such as walking. By adopting a health-promoting life-style, you can do much to slow the natural process of physical decline. Another important area in which you can gain control is health awareness. By being alert to early warning signs of disease, you are more likely to avoid illness and stay fit and healthy.

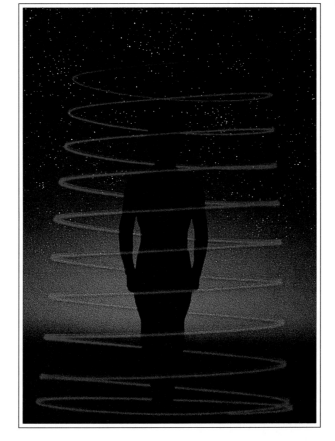

HEALTH AND LIFE EXPECTANCY

How can we truly measure health? For each of us, one entirely subjective indicator of health is how we feel, both physically and emotionally. But the age at which people die is precisely measurable and provides a good indication of the health of the population as a whole. Today, fewer people are dying as young as they did 100 years ago, confirming that major improvements in health have been accomplished.

Longevity is not the only measure of health. Health is reflected in the physical state of our body systems, our ability to withstand infection, and our growing ability to expand our physical prowess – best seen today at major athletic events where world records regularly topple.

Life expectancies: Men
The graph below shows how life expectancies at birth for men in the US have changed in this century. Compare these figures with life expectancies for women in the graph opposite.

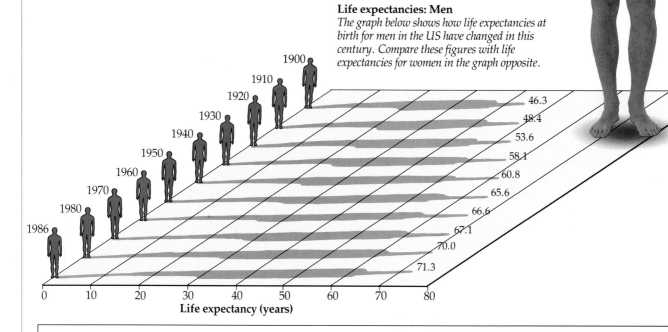

1900 — 46.3
1910 — 48.4
1920 — 53.6
1930 — 58.1
1940 — 60.8
1950 — 65.6
1960 — 66.6
1970 — 67.1
1980 — 70.0
1986 — 71.3

Life expectancy (years)
0   10   20   30   40   50   60   70   80

AGE AND LIFE EXPECTANCY

Strange as it may seem, your life expectancy increases as you get older. The key is to stay alive. Even a 100-year-old man can expect to live a few years, despite the fact that his life expectancy would have been just over 40 years at the time of his birth.

The numbers game
The chart shows the age to which people of different age groups in the US can expect to live at the present time. Figures given are averages; individual life expectancy depends on many factors, including heredity, environment, and life-style.

Present age	WHITE		BLACK	
	Men	Women	Men	Women
20	73.4	79.9	67.3	75.3
30	74.2	80.1	68.5	75.7
40	74.9	80.5	70.3	76.6
50	76.1	81.2	72.7	78.0
60	78.2	82.6	76.1	80.3
70	81.7	85.1	80.8	83.9
80	86.9	88.8	86.8	88.5
85	90.1	91.4	90.5	91.7

Health can also be measured by the quality of our lives over an increasing number of years. Today "the golden years" can be a term with real meaning.

For most of human history, the average life expectancy was between 30 and 40 years. However, in developed countries, most people now live beyond 70. The major factors that account for people living longer in developed countries are reforms in sanitation (such as pure water supplies and safe disposal of sewage and trash) and adequate nutrition in childhood, along with advances in medical care – especially the development of vaccines and antibiotics.

Eventually, with continued advancement, most people will live out their genetically determined life span. Human beings will always vary – in height, intelligence, or artistic and athletic ability – and their genetically determined life spans will vary too. Just as being tall or having red hair tends to run in families, so does having a long (or short) life span. The ideal would be for most people to live a full 80 to 90 years, with a minimum of disease and disability.

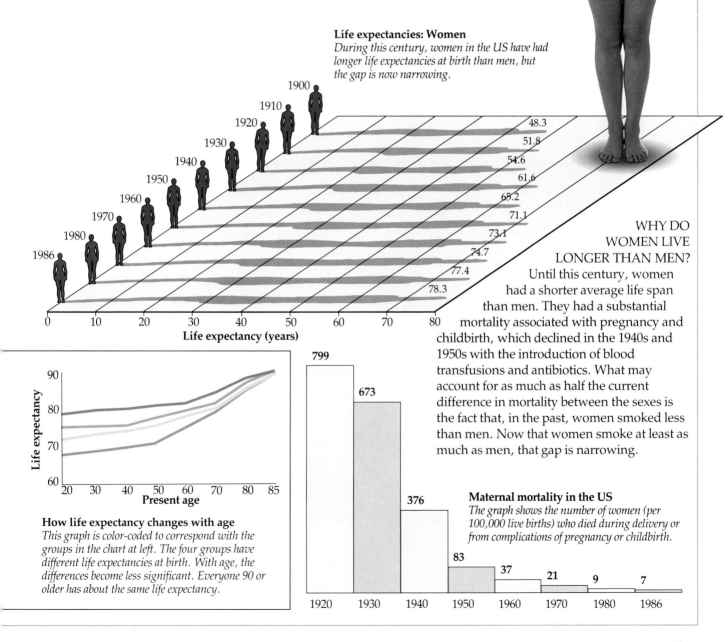

Life expectancies: Women
During this century, women in the US have had longer life expectancies at birth than men, but the gap is now narrowing.

1900 — 48.3
1910 — 51.8
1920 — 54.6
1930 — 61.6
1940 — 65.2
1950 — 71.1
1960 — 73.1
1970 — 74.7
1980 — 77.4
1986 — 78.3

Life expectancy (years)

WHY DO WOMEN LIVE LONGER THAN MEN?
Until this century, women had a shorter average life span than men. They had a substantial mortality associated with pregnancy and childbirth, which declined in the 1940s and 1950s with the introduction of blood transfusions and antibiotics. What may account for as much as half the current difference in mortality between the sexes is the fact that, in the past, women smoked less than men. Now that women smoke at least as much as men, that gap is narrowing.

How life expectancy changes with age
This graph is color-coded to correspond with the groups in the chart at left. The four groups have different life expectancies at birth. With age, the differences become less significant. Everyone 90 or older has about the same life expectancy.

799
673
376
83
37
21
9
7

1920 1930 1940 1950 1960 1970 1980 1986

Maternal mortality in the US
The graph shows the number of women (per 100,000 live births) who died during delivery or from complications of pregnancy or childbirth.

LIFE EXPECTANCY AROUND THE WORLD

Only in Western Europe, North America, Japan, Australia, and New Zealand can most people expect to survive into old age. In other continents and countries, childhood deaths remain common, although vaccination programs and more effective treatment for diarrheal diseases are reducing the numbers. Deaths from infections such as tuberculosis and from parasitic diseases such as schistosomiasis strike adults in their most productive years.

Theoretically, the high mortality among children and young adults in developing countries contributes to rapid population growth. People who depend on their children for support are not likely to limit the number of children they have until they are confident that most will survive.

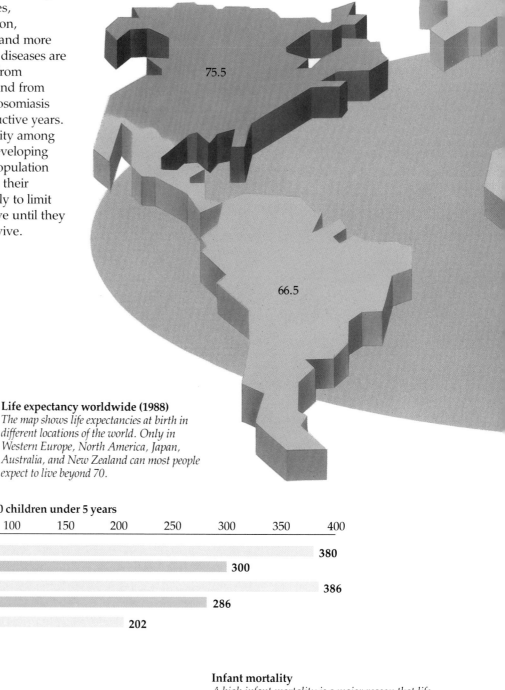

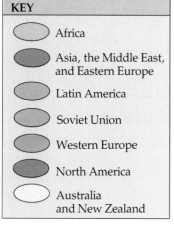

KEY

- Africa
- Asia, the Middle East, and Eastern Europe
- Latin America
- Soviet Union
- Western Europe
- North America
- Australia and New Zealand

Life expectancy worldwide (1988)
The map shows life expectancies at birth in different locations of the world. Only in Western Europe, North America, Japan, Australia, and New Zealand can most people expect to live beyond 70.

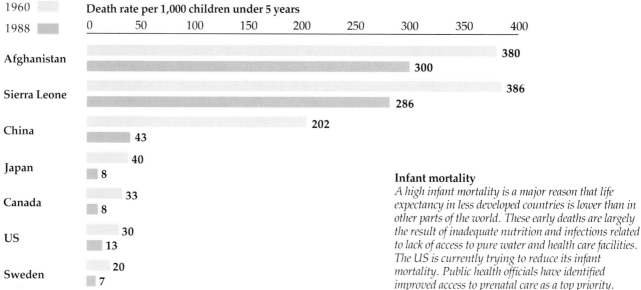

1960

Death rate per 1,000 children under 5 years

1988

	0	50	100	150	200	250	300	350	400

Afghanistan 380 / 300

Sierra Leone 386 / 286

China 202 / 43

Japan 40 / 8

Canada 33 / 8

US 30 / 13

Sweden 20 / 7

Infant mortality
A high infant mortality is a major reason that life expectancy in less developed countries is lower than in other parts of the world. These early deaths are largely the result of inadequate nutrition and infections related to lack of access to pure water and health care facilities. The US is currently trying to reduce its infant mortality. Public health officials have identified improved access to prenatal care as a top priority.

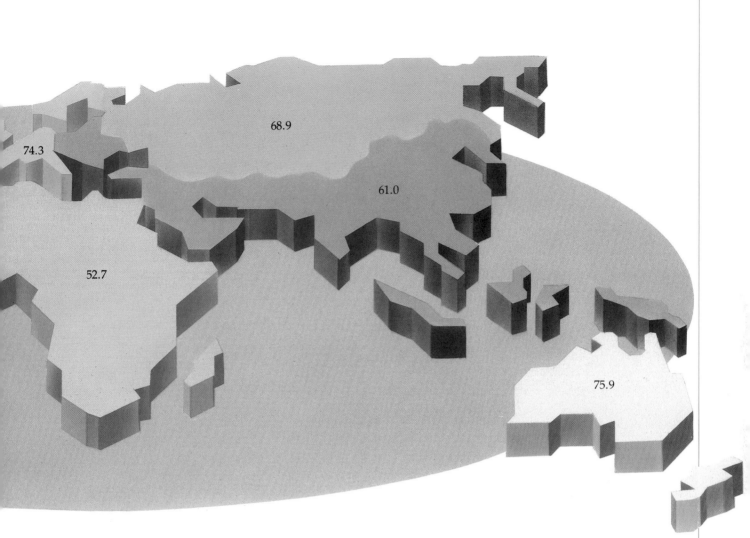

74.3

68.9

61.0

52.7

75.9

WHERE IS THE LAND OF LONGEVITY?

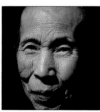

If you want to live to an old age, your chances are best if you were born in and live in Japan. Life expectancy at birth there is the longest in the world at 78 years (in 1988). The healthy Japanese diet, which is diverse and extremely low in fat, is thought to be a contributing factor. Anecdotal reports exist of isolated societies elsewhere, often in mountainous areas of the world, that have extraordinarily long-lived populations. While these claims offer some basis for intriguing speculation and research, they usually cannot be substantiated with reliable birth and death data.

WHO HAS THE SHORTEST LIFE SPAN?

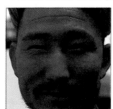

People born in Sierra Leone or Ethiopia in Africa have a life expectancy at birth of only 41 years (in 1988) – the shortest in the world. Natives of Afghanistan and Guinea have the next shortest life expectancy – 42 years at birth. Such yearly figures are always slightly misleading because they reflect singular circumstances such as the drought, famine, and attendant epidemics in Ethiopia or the prolonged war in Afghanistan. However, apart from these exceptional occurrences, a high infant mortality is usually a major factor accounting for a short life expectancy.

HEALTH – CHANCE OR CHOICE?

Many different factors determine how healthy we will be throughout our lives. Some are genetic and some are the result of environmental influences. Others have to do with our individual habits and activities and the emotional stresses and pressures in our lives.

EFFECT OF HEREDITY AND ENVIRONMENT

Some people are born genetically predisposed to certain illnesses, or they are born genetically programmed to have a shorter-than-average life expectancy. However, in most cases, there is little biological basis for variations in health among individuals.

Studies have shown that socioeconomic differences have a pervasive effect on health. These differences are environmental, not genetic; they are associated with poor housing, inadequate nutrition, and lack of access to immunization programs. Because of such factors, the

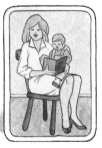

Factors beyond your control
Your genes, the socioeconomic environment into which you are born, and early psychological or emotional experiences – factors you cannot control – all influence your future health.

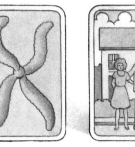

children of parents working in unskilled occupations are less healthy than those of skilled workers and professionals.

PSYCHOLOGICAL INFLUENCES

Within any defined social or occupational grouping, susceptibility to illness varies. Psychological stresses, however, seem to increase the likelihood of both minor and major physical illnesses, from the common cold to peptic ulcer. In the work environment, repeated absences because of sickness are clearly associated with financial anxieties, marital problems, or serious illness in another member of

How old are your grandparents?
If you want to live 90 years or longer you need to be lucky – the most important factor is out of your control. Longevity is largely determined by heredity. People whose parents and grandparents lived past the age of 90 are likely to do the same. A person whose parents or grandparents did not live beyond 80 is unlikely to live much longer than that.

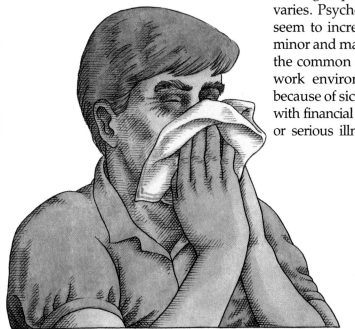

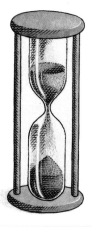

Why do some people get more colds than others?
People who have school-age children tend to catch colds more frequently just because they are exposed to more cold viruses. But any person's chances of contracting a cold are increased if he or she is under psychological or emotional stress.

the family. And it is negative stress that damages health. The employee passed over for a promotion is more likely to become sick than his or her colleague who is given the new job, even if there are increased responsibilities and demands associated with the promotion.

WHAT YOU CAN DO

Although you cannot change your background and cannot always avoid psychological stress, you have control over significant choices of life-style. You can make decisions about how much exercise you get, your diet, habits such as smoking and drinking, the risks you take in your sexual activity, and the extent to which you make an effort to prevent accidents.

You can't reprogram your genes, but you can help yourself by learning about any family disorders, telling your doctor about them, and having appropriate checkups. You also can be aware of your body and how it functions. If you know what is normal, such as how often you have a bowel movement, you are more likely to notice change that might indicate a problem. When you report these changes to your doctor, you increase your chances of prompt, effective treatment.

Safety sense
Statistics show that accident rates are highest for people from 15 to 24 years old. The rates climb again after age 65. You can prevent most accidents by taking precautions such as using a seat belt when you drive or wearing a helmet if you ride a motorcycle.

Taking control
By adopting a healthy life-style, increasing your awareness of risk factors, and being alert to possible indications of sickness, you will reduce your chances of premature death and improve the quality of your life by staying healthy longer.

A healthy life-style
Regular exercise and a varied, balanced diet are the cornerstones of good health. Smoking, excessive drinking, and other forms of drug abuse are destructive. You can also protect yourself against high-risk sexual activities.

15

STAY ON TOP OF YOUR HEALTH

One of the main objectives of monitoring your health and of having regular checkups is to detect diseases early.

For some diseases – such as cancers of the breast, skin, testicle, or colon – early detection can make the difference between cure and serious illness or death. Some of these diseases may make themselves known by a variety of symptoms; it is important to be alert to the symptoms you need to take seriously. Other disorders, such as hypertension, high cholesterol, and cervical cancer, may be largely symptomless, but your doctor can perform a screening test that can detect them at an early stage.

Is it flu?
Most people who have a fever, a sore throat, and muscular aches and pains have a viral infection (flu). Call your doctor if you have other symptoms (see page 18).

WHEN EARLY DIAGNOSIS IS VITAL

For some acute, infectious diseases, diagnosis within the first 24 hours can be lifesaving. One example is bacterial meningitis (inflammation of the membranes that cover the brain). Many other infections, ranging from acute appendicitis to syphilis, also require prompt diagnosis. Of the noninfectious diseases for which timely action is needed, the most important are high blood pressure, coronary heart disease, and cancer. Millions of lives have been prolonged by the recognition and treatment of symptomless high blood pressure. Many types of cancer are curable if detected at an early stage. Your awareness of

Take care of yourself
Many health organizations distribute excellent pamphlets that give helpful medical information and details of what to expect from your doctor.

FRY NOW. PAY LATER.

AMERICAN CANCER SOCIETY

1989

Año Europeo de Información sobre el Cáncer

15% MENOS DE VICTIMAS EN EL AÑO 2000

Cáncer

MONTHLY DO-IT-YOURSELF CHECKUPS

Skin self-examination
Men and women of all ages should examine their skin for signs of skin cancer. These signs include any new or existing mole that darkens, itches, bleeds, or grows. Another sign is any sore that will not heal, especially on a part of the body exposed to the sun. If you have been exposed to the sun for long periods, examine yourself with extra care.

Breast self-examination
Examination of your breasts is an excellent way to detect a change in their shape and to feel for any lumps that might be early signs of cancer. All women should begin self-examination at age 20. Examine yourself at the end of each menstrual period. After the menopause, examine your breasts on the same day of each month.

Testicle self-examination
Men should do this examination to detect lumps or swellings that could be an early sign of testicular cancer. Starting at age 20, examine your testicles monthly, ideally during or after a warm bath or shower.

HEALTH CHECKUPS BY MEDICAL PROFESSIONALS

These recommendations are not absolute. Your age and previous medical problems will determine the frequency with which you need specific tests.

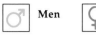 ♂ Men ♀ Women

EYE EXAMINATION
 To detect any visual defects or eye muscle disorders and to look for any signs of disease.
At high risk Anyone diagnosed as having diabetes or high blood pressure or who has a family history of glaucoma.

DENTAL CHECKUP
To check on the health of the teeth, gums, tongue, and mouth and to look for oral cancer.
At high risk Tobacco smokers or chewers.

CERVICAL (PAP) SMEAR
 To detect abnormal cells in the cervical lining that could develop into cancer.
At high risk Women already diagnosed and treated for precancerous changes or for herpes or genital warts.

MEASUREMENT OF BLOOD PRESSURE
 To detect high blood pressure at an early stage, before complications develop.
At high risk Anyone with a family history of hypertension, heart or kidney disease, or stroke or diabetes, or who is overweight or taking oral contraceptives.

BLOOD CHOLESTEROL TEST
 To detect people at high risk of coronary heart disease.
At high risk Anyone with a family history of early-onset coronary heart disease.

MAMMOGRAPHY (BREAST X-RAY)
 To detect breast cancer early, before it can be detected by physical examination.
At high risk Anyone with a close relative who has had cancer.

EXAMINATION OF THE RECTUM AND COLON
To detect cancer of the rectum and colon. There are three separate tests – a) digital rectal examination, b) tests for hidden blood in the stool, and c) sigmoidoscopy.
At high risk Anyone with an immediate family member who has had cancer of the colon or rectum; polyps of the colon; or long-standing, extensive ulcerative colitis.

COMPLETE PHYSICAL EXAMINATION
 To determine your health status and develop your relationship with your doctor.

TEST	FREQUENCY	
	NOT AT HIGH RISK	**AT HIGH RISK**
TEENAGERS TO AGE 30		
♂ ♀	Every 2 years if you have problems with your vision.	At least once a year.
♂ ♀	Every 6 months until age 21, then at least once a year.	As your dentist recommends.
♀	Annually for women over 18 and all sexually active women, or as your doctor recommends.	Annually.
♂ ♀	Begin at age 20; after 20, at 3- to 5-year intervals.	Annually.
♂ ♀	At the time of your first physical examination.	If abnormal, follow your doctor's advice.
♂ ♀	Usually not necessary.	a) Annually after age 20.
♂ ♀	Twice in your 20s.	
ADULTS 30 TO 50		
♂ ♀	Every 2 years. If you have good vision, start at 40.	About once a year.
♂ ♀	At least once a year.	As your dentist recommends.
♀	Every 1 to 3 years.	Annually.
♂ ♀	Every 3 to 5 years.	Annually.
♂ ♀	Depends on results of last test. If normal, repeat in 3 to 5 years.	If abnormal, follow your doctor's advice.
♀	Once between 35 and 40; every 1 to 2 years between 40 and 50.	Every 1 to 2 years, beginning at age 35.
♂ ♀	a) Annually after 40.	a) Annually. b) Annually. c) Every 3 to 5 years.
♂ ♀	Every 1 to 2 years, as your doctor recommends.	
ADULTS 50 AND OVER		
♂ ♀	Every 2 years.	At least once a year.
♂ ♀	Every 1 to 2 years.	As your dentist recommends.
♀	Every 3 to 5 years.	Annually.
♂ ♀	Annually.	As your doctor recommends.
♂ ♀	Depends on results of last test. If normal, repeat in 3 to 5 years.	If abnormal, follow your doctor's advice.
♀	Annually.	Same as for those not at high risk.
♂ ♀	a) Annually. b) Annually. c) Every 3 to 5 years.	Same as for those not at high risk.
♂ ♀	Every 1 to 2 years to age 65; after 65, every year.	

early symptoms and signs, which you may detect during self-examination, is also a significant means of discovering cancer at an early, treatable stage.

Some noninfectious conditions, including ectopic pregnancy and intestinal obstruction, may be fatal without immediate treatment. Early diagnosis is also important for glaucoma, which does not produce symptoms until an advanced stage.

CANCER WARNING SIGNS

If you notice any of the following early symptoms of cancer, contact your doctor immediately:
- Sore that does not heal
- Persistent cough or hoarseness
- Unusual or newly developed indigestion or difficult or painful swallowing
- Obvious change in a wart or mole
- Lump in breast or elsewhere
- Change in bowel or bladder habits
- Unusual bleeding or discharge

TWO IMPORTANT REMINDERS

1 Do not ignore symptoms that could be early indicators of a serious condition. Call your doctor immediately if you see the following signs of trouble.

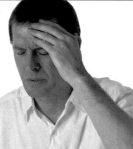

Sudden onset of a high temperature, shaking chills, vomiting, diarrhea, headache
These are symptoms of blood poisoning. They occur when the bloodstream is invaded by viruses, bacteria, or toxins.

Red eye, blurred vision, severe pain
A person with these symptoms could have a type of glaucoma that must be treated immediately to avoid permanent damage to vision.

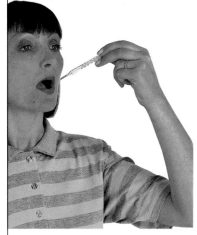

Raised temperature, drowsiness, stiff neck
A child or adult with a high fever, who is drowsy or won't wake up, who complains about bright lights or a stiff neck, and who might also have a rash could have meningitis.

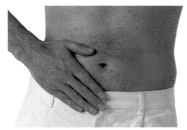

Severe abdominal pain
Abdominal pain that is not temporarily relieved by vomiting or that persists for more than 6 hours could indicate an inflammation or obstruction in the abdominal area.

Persistent, painless sore or ulcer
A painless sore on or around the genitals, in the mouth, or on the fingers may be the first sign of syphilis or cancer.

2 Remember that your doctor is the one who should diagnose serious disorders.

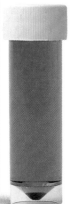

Abrupt onset of dark brown urine
Dark brown urine could indicate that the flow of bile from the liver is obstructed, a cause of jaundice.

CASE HISTORY
AN ITCHY ROUND RASH

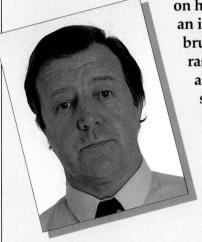

JOHN, A MARINE BIOLOGIST in Massachusetts, is an avid backpacker in his spare time. Several days after a weekend in the woods, he noticed a slightly itchy red rash on his calf, which he thought was an insect bite or the result of a brush with poison ivy. The rash was distinctly circular and did not clear up after several days. John decided to check with his doctor.

PERSONAL DETAILS
Name John Rice
Age 52
Occupation Marine biologist
Family John is married and has no children.

MEDICAL BACKGROUND
John has never had any serious illnesses and he believes he is in good physical condition.

THE CONSULTATION
By the time John visits his doctor, he has missed several days of work because he feels feverish and fatigued, and some of his muscles and joints hurt. He complains about dizziness, chills, and a stiff neck as well. His rash has persisted and has a whitish center. John's doctor asks him if he noticed a tick on his skin at any time. John says that by the time he thought to examine his skin specifically for a tick he could not find one.

FURTHER INVESTIGATION
The doctor takes a blood sample. John's blood shows antibodies to the bacteria that cause Lyme disease. They are transmitted through the bite of the tick that is the carrier. (If the first test result had been negative, the doctor might have asked John to return for additional tests in a week or so to ensure that the results were accurate.)

THE DIAGNOSIS
The doctor confirms that John has the widely publicized though uncommon infection called LYME DISEASE. He says that the tick may have been attached for several hours, without John feeling a thing. He assures John that, at this early stage, the disease is easily treatable. If left untreated, Lyme disease can cause a debilitating heart disorder, muscle weakness, arthritis, and meningitis (an inflammation of the membranes covering the brain and spinal cord).

THE TREATMENT
John is relieved to learn that the organism is sensitive to many antibiotics (including penicillin, erythromycin, tetracycline, and cefotaxime). His doctor prescribes tetracycline, which John takes for about 3 weeks.

THE FOLLOW-UP
All of John's symptoms disappear, and he recovers completely with no complications. John is glad that he paid close attention to the rash on his leg and other symptoms and sought medical attention early. Now when he goes backpacking or spends any long period of time outdoors, he wears long pants and tucks them into his socks. He uses an insect repellent, and he checks carefully for ticks on his skin during the spring and summer months.

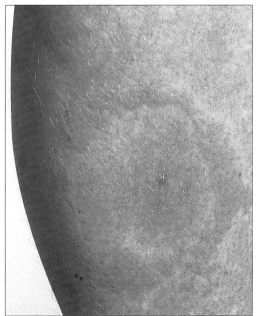

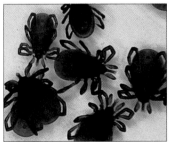

The doctor's examination
The rash that accompanies acute Lyme disease (shown at left) is red, but as it enlarges it forms a white center. The rash often develops at the site of the tick bite. Deer ticks (shown below, magnified ×3) transmit the bacteria that cause Lyme disease. The ticks usually live on deer but may infest pets.

CHAPTER TWO

MONITOR YOUR PHYSICAL HEALTH

WHEN WE GREET each other by saying "How are you today?" we are expressing interest in the commonplace ups and downs that we all experience. Factors such as the weather, last night's sleep, how much or what we have had to eat, whether today's events are tedious or exciting, and our interactions with family and colleagues all help determine how good we feel each day.

You are likely to feel on top of the world only if your physical health is good. Keeping your body in good shape requires that you establish healthy habits, including a well-balanced diet, regular exercise, and control or avoidance of stress to the extent possible. Some people use middle age as a reason to abandon any attempt to stay in shape. If you are healthy there is little excuse for not being in good physical condition.

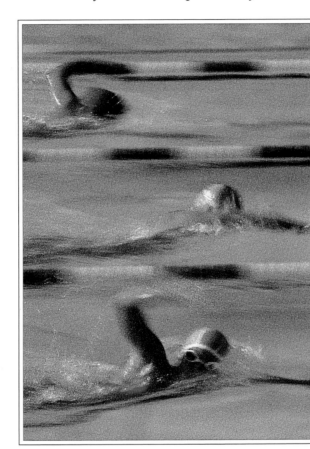

In this chapter we explain how to assess your heart, lungs, and muscles to find out just how physically fit you are. Your health is also closely linked with your diet. The availability of a wide variety of nutritious foods is one of the main reasons people today live longer. But you have more choices to make than ever before. You can substantially improve your health by making a habit of choosing fresh fruits and vegetables, grains, fish, and lean meats, and cutting back on high-fat foods. We offer ideas on how you can make these important food choices without going hungry or feeling deprived at mealtimes. At any age it is important to stay in good shape and to detect any signs of disease at an early, treatable stage. One important step is to have regular medical checkups with your doctor. However, you can and should monitor your health between these checkups. You are in the best position to detect changes that your doctor should know about. Learn to know your body and how it functions under day-to-day circumstances. Be alert to changes in these patterns and learn what signs to look for and what symptoms to report to your doctor and you will have taken the first step toward lasting good health. In this chapter we tell you how to monitor your health from day to day as well as under special circumstances, such as pregnancy. We also address the needs of people who have conditions such as diabetes or hypertension and who may need to perform more specialized tests regularly at home. Whatever your state of health, the specific information you can gather about your condition may help guide you in your own health practices.

HOW FIT ARE YOU?

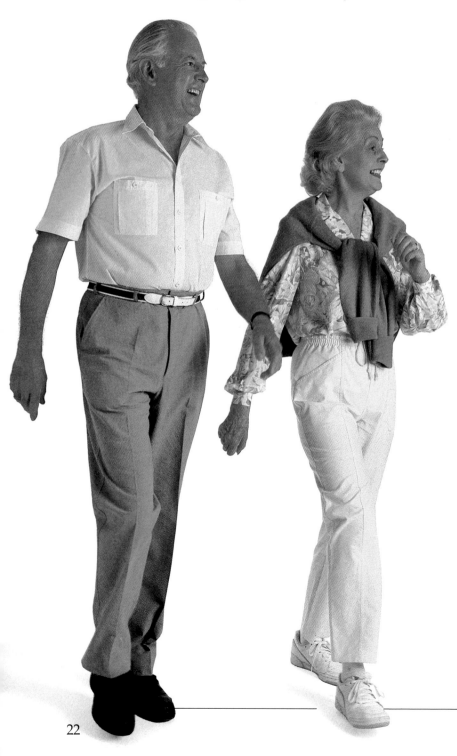

STUDIES CLEARLY SHOW that being physically fit increases your chances of staying healthy and living longer. How do you know whether you are fit? The most accurate measurements of fitness are carried out in an exercise physiology laboratory. But you can do some simple tests, such as the 1-mile walking test explained at right, to get a general idea of your level of fitness.

Fitness consists of three components – strength (the ability to carry, lift, push, or pull a heavy load), flexibility (the ability to bend, stretch, and twist), and endurance (the ability to maintain effort for an extended period of time). Endurance is the most important indicator of your general health because it reflects the efficiency of your heart and lungs.

EVALUATING YOUR FITNESS

No single measurement of performance classifies you as fit or unfit. Just seeing how well you do at everyday activities will give you some idea. If you become breathless after climbing a flight of stairs or hurrying to catch a bus, you clearly could benefit from some conditioning. Check with your doctor before you start an exercise program.

Walking to fitness
The long-term effects of moderate exercise, such as walking several times a week, are significant in terms of increasing fitness levels and lowering death rates. Walking is a form of exercise that can be easily incorporated into anyone's life. Experts recommend 30 to 40 minutes of brisk walking (at about 4 miles per hour) at least three times a week to obtain significant benefit. However, even walking for shorter periods once or twice a week is better than no exercise at all. You can use the 1-mile walking test (opposite page) as a simple method of assessing your level of fitness. You can repeat the test at intervals of a few weeks during your fitness improvement program to measure your progress.

DO THE 1-MILE WALKING TEST

PREPARING FOR THE TEST

♦ Complete the PHYSICAL ACTIVITY READINESS QUESTIONNAIRE (right). If you answer "yes" to any question, talk to your doctor before taking the test. Also check the list of medications (below right). If you are taking any of those listed, the test is not valid for you.

♦ Use a stopwatch or a watch with a second hand to time yourself and to measure your pulse rate after the test.

♦ You will want to record your time and pulse rate. You need these figures to determine your fitness level.

♦ Wear a comfortable pair of shoes.

♦ A flat quarter-mile track or an indoor track is the best setting for the test. If you do not live near a track, use your car to measure a distance of 1 mile on a flat road that has little traffic.

♦ If you are walking outside, do not take the test when weather conditions are extremely hot, cold, wet, or windy.

♦ Do not eat for 2 hours and do not smoke or drink caffeinated beverages for 3 hours before the test.

♦ Spend at least 5 minutes warming up before the test. Do some stretching exercises and walk slowly.

♦ It is normal to perspire and breathe heavily during any exercise session. It is also normal for your heart to beat faster during exercise. However, if you experience any of the following symptoms, stop exercising and seek medical attention promptly:

♦ Persistent pain or pressure in your chest, shoulder, arm, neck, or jaw
♦ Nausea or dizziness
♦ Skipped heartbeats

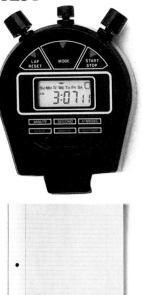

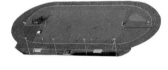

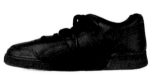

PHYSICAL ACTIVITY READINESS QUESTIONNAIRE

♦ Has your doctor ever told you that you have heart trouble?   YES/NO
♦ Do you frequently have pains in your heart region and/or your chest?   YES/NO
♦ Do you frequently feel dizzy or have spells of severe dizziness?   YES/NO
♦ Has a doctor ever told you that your blood pressure was too high?   YES/NO
♦ Do you have any bone or joint condition, such as arthritis, that might be aggravated by exercise?   YES/NO
♦ Is there a good physical reason not mentioned here why you could not participate in an exercise program, even if you wanted to?   YES/NO
♦ Are you over 65 and not accustomed to regular exercise?   YES/NO

MEDICATIONS

Some drugs prevent the heart rate from increasing during exercise or cause it to increase above normal levels. The walking test is not valid if you are taking any of the following:

Alpha blockers
Beta blockers
Bronchodilators
Calcium channel blockers
Centrally acting adrenergic inhibitors
Cold medications
Diet medications
Major tranquilizers
Nitrates
Nonadrenergic peripheral vasodilators
Peripheral acting adrenergic inhibitors
Thyroid medications
Tricyclic antidepressants

TAKING THE TEST

1 After warming up for 5 minutes, walk briskly for 1 mile at a steady pace. If you are using a quarter-mile track, walk the four laps using the inside lane.

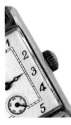

2 Use your watch or stopwatch to determine your time in minutes and seconds.

3 Immediately after recording your time, stop and take your pulse for exactly 15 seconds and record this number. To take your pulse, put your second and third fingers together and place them on the inside of your wrist or place the heel of your right hand directly over your heart. Practice taking your pulse before the test so that you will be able to find it easily and quickly to get an accurate count after the test. Immediacy is important because the heart rate decreases quickly.

4 After you have recorded your 15-second pulse, continue to walk slowly for at least 5 minutes to allow your heart rate and blood pressure to return to normal.

5 Now assess your current fitness level by consulting the chart on page 24.

HOW DID YOU SCORE?

1 To convert the 15-second pulse count (that you took immediately after walking the mile) into your pulse rate in beats per minute, multiply the count by 4. For example, if your 15-second pulse count was 32 beats, your pulse rate was 32 × 4, or 128 beats per minute.

2 Read down the far left-hand column in the chart below until you come to your age category. Find your pulse rate from the walking test in the column titled PULSE RATE within your age category. (If you do not find your exact pulse rate in the column, round it off to the nearest 10. For example, a pulse rate of 122 would be rounded off to 120, or a pulse rate of 138 would be rounded off to 140.) Then, reading horizontally in the appropriate columns under MEN and WOMEN, determine whether your 1-mile walk time falls in the MEDIUM FITNESS or HIGH FITNESS category.

3 For every 10 pounds over 175 pounds that you weigh if you are a man, or every 10 pounds over 125 pounds if you are a woman, you must walk 15 seconds faster to qualify for a fitness category. For every 10 pounds under 175 pounds that you weigh if you are a man, or every 10 pounds under 125 pounds if you are a woman, you can walk 15 seconds slower to qualify for a fitness category.

AGE	PULSE RATE	MEN		WOMEN	
		MEDIUM FITNESS	HIGH FITNESS	MEDIUM FITNESS	HIGH FITNESS
20	110	17:06 to 19:36	Less than 17:06	19:08 to 20:57	Less than 19:08
to	120	16:36 to 19:10	Less than 16:36	18:38 to 20:27	Less than 18:38
29	130	16:06 to 18:35	Less than 16:06	18:12 to 20:00	Less than 18:12
	140	15:36 to 18:06	Less than 15:36	17:42 to 19:30	Less than 17:42
	150	15:10 to 17:36	Less than 15:10	17:12 to 19:00	Less than 17:12
	160	14:42 to 17:09	Less than 14:42	16:42 to 18:30	Less than 16:42
	170	14:12 to 16:39	Less than 14:12	16:12 to 18:00	Less than 16:12
30	110	15:54 to 18:21	Less than 15:54	17:52 to 19:46	Less than 17:52
to	120	15:24 to 17:52	Less than 15:24	17:24 to 19:18	Less than 17:24
39	130	14:54 to 17:22	Less than 14:54	16:54 to 18:48	Less than 16:54
	140	14:30 to 16:54	Less than 14:30	16:24 to 18:18	Less than 16:24
	150	14:00 to 16:26	Less than 14:00	15:54 to 17:48	Less than 15:54
	160	13:30 to 15:58	Less than 13:30	15:24 to 17:18	Less than 15:24
	170	13:01 to 15:28	Less than 13:01	14:55 to 16:54	Less than 14:55
40	110	15:38 to 18:05	Less than 15:38	17:20 to 19:15	Less than 17:20
to	120	15:09 to 17:36	Less than 15:09	16:50 to 18:45	Less than 16:50
49	130	14:41 to 17:07	Less than 14:41	16:24 to 18:18	Less than 16:24
	140	14:12 to 16:38	Less than 14:12	15:54 to 17:48	Less than 15:54
	150	13:42 to 16:09	Less than 13:42	15:24 to 17:18	Less than 15:24
	160	13:15 to 15:42	Less than 13:15	14:54 to 16:48	Less than 14:54
	170	12:45 to 15:12	Less than 12:45	14:25 to 16:18	Less than 14:25
50	110	15:22 to 17:49	Less than 15:22	17:04 to 18:40	Less than 17:04
to	120	14:53 to 17:20	Less than 14:53	16:36 to 18:12	Less than 16:36
59	130	14:24 to 16:51	Less than 14:24	16:06 to 17:42	Less than 16:06
	140	13:51 to 16:22	Less than 13:51	15:36 to 17:18	Less than 15:36
	150	13:26 to 15:53	Less than 13:26	15:06 to 16:48	Less than 15:06
	160	12:59 to 15:26	Less than 12:59	14:36 to 16:18	Less than 14:36
	170	12:30 to 14:56	Less than 12:30	14:06 to 15:48	Less than 14:06
60	110	15:33 to 17:55	Less than 15:33	16:36 to 18:00	Less than 16:36
and	120	15:04 to 17:24	Less than 15:04	16:06 to 17:30	Less than 16:06
over	130	14:36 to 16:57	Less than 14:36	15:37 to 17:01	Less than 15:37
	140	14:07 to 16:28	Less than 14:07	15:09 to 16:31	Less than 15:09
	150	13:39 to 15:59	Less than 13:39	14:39 to 16:02	Less than 14:39
	160	13:10 to 15:30	Less than 13:10	14:12 to 15:32	Less than 14:12
	170	12:42 to 15:04	Less than 12:42	13:42 to 15:04	Less than 13:42

4 You may notice that, as a person ages, for a given pulse rate, he or she must walk faster to qualify for a fitness category. As we age, our maximal pulse rate decreases. A 20-year-old person who is exercising at a pulse rate of 110 beats per minute is capable of getting his or her pulse rate as high as 200 beats per minute during strenuous exercise. A person who is 60 years old who is exercising at a pulse rate of 110 beats per minute is capable of getting his or her pulse rate to only about 160 beats per minute. Thus, for any given pulse rate, a younger person is working at a lower percentage of maximum than an older person.

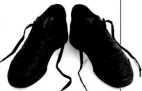

RISKS OF EXCESS WEIGHT

People who carry a greater load of body fat put extra stress on their heart, lungs, and joints. Being overweight or obese (usually defined as being 20 percent or more over the maximum desirable weight for your height) increases your risk of high blood pressure, diabetes, and high cholesterol, all of which increase your risk of coronary heart disease. The added stress on your joints from being overweight can aggravate arthritic conditions and lead to greater disability later in life.

Regular exercise should be an essential part of your lifelong fitness plan because it can help reduce body fat, develop your muscle mass and maintain its tone, and prevent disease. Exercising regularly can also give you a psychological lift. Check to see if your weight falls into the normal range for your height by referring to the table on page 139.

WAIST-TO-HIP RATIO

For someone who is overweight, the risk of heart disease depends in part on where the fat is stored. For reasons that are still not fully understood, the risk of heart disease is greater for a person whose body fat is concentrated in the abdominal area, rather than in the hips and thighs. The measure of this factor is your waist-to-hip ratio. To calculate the ratio, measure your waist and your hip circumferences, then divide your waist measurement by your hip measurement.

What do the results mean?

Men who have a waist-to-hip ratio higher than 1.0 and women who have a ratio higher than 0.8 have a greater accumulation of fat in the abdominal area and are at greater risk of heart disease. A recent study suggests that an average person with more fat around the hips has a higher level of a protective form of cholesterol (high-density lipoprotein) than a person who has more fat in the abdominal area.

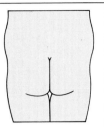

Barrel shape
Someone with a high waist-to-hip ratio – a barrel shape or pot belly – is at a higher risk of heart disease.

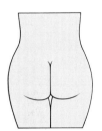

Pear shape
Someone with a low waist-to-hip ratio – a pear-shaped body – is at a lower risk of heart disease.

HOW ABOUT SWIMMING FOR FITNESS?

If you don't like to walk or jog, swimming is an excellent alternative form of aerobic exercise. Studies have shown that it takes 12 to 20 weeks, swimming a minimum of 3 days a week, to improve your cardiovascular fitness. Alternating days of training with rest days gives your body time to recover. Even swimming once a week will improve your fitness, and you may enjoy the relaxing effects of being in the water.

A good workout does not mean swimming as fast as you can for as long as you can – that could be dangerous and would not improve your fitness much. You can plan your workouts, with the help of a book or an instructor, to gradually increase your level of fitness. Each workout should consist of a

Your target heart rate
Take your pulse after the main set of each workout. To improve your cardiovascular fitness, you should aim for a target heart rate during each main set. Your target rate should be about 70 percent of your maximum heart rate. Calculate your maximum heart rate by subtracting your age from 220 beats per minute.

warm-up (some stretching exercises, kicking at the side of the pool, or slowly swimming a few lengths), a main set (a planned number of strokes, repeated several times with intervening 1-minute rest periods), and a cool-down (treading water, swimming some slow, relaxed lengths, or doing stretching exercises). During the main sets of your successive workouts, you should swim progressively greater distances.

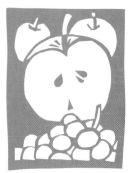

HOW HEALTHY IS YOUR DIET?

A HEALTHY DIET CONTAINS the widest possible variety of natural foods. It provides you with a good balance of carbohydrates, fat, protein, vitamins, minerals, and fiber. In general, the amount of food energy (calories) supplied by your diet should not exceed the amount of energy you expend, so that your weight remains relatively constant over time.

The primary dietary problem for many people living in developed countries is that they consume more food than they need. Because they are eating too much, these people almost certainly get enough carbohydrates, fat, and pro-tein. However, if their diet does not contain enough whole grains, green leafy vegetables, and fruits, they may not be getting a sufficient amount of vitamins, minerals, or fiber. Improving your diet doesn't mean cutting out fat

HOW POOR EATING HABITS CAN AFFECT YOUR HEALTH

Sometimes you can eat indulgently without significantly affecting your health. However, if your diet consistently lacks vital elements, includes excessive amounts of some foods, or exceeds your energy requirements, one or more of the following health problems could develop.

Increased risk of cancer
A high intake of alcohol or of smoked or salt-cured foods may increase the risk of some cancers. High-fat diets have also been associated with a greater incidence of certain types of cancer.

Weight gain and obesity
If you consistently consume more calories than you expend through physical activity, the surplus calories will be stored as body fat. Overweight people are at an increased risk for a number of disorders, including diabetes, high blood pressure, elevated cholesterol level, coronary heart disease, stroke, and gallstones.

Heart disease and stroke
A high intake of fat, particularly saturated fats (animal fat, butter, and whole milk and cream), contributes to the development of atherosclerosis (narrowing of arteries by the accumulation of fatty deposits). Atherosclerosis is the main cause of coronary heart disease, peripheral vascular disease, and stroke.

High blood pressure
Many people take in more sodium, in the form of added salt or sodium-containing foods, than they need. Reduced salt intake has been shown to benefit some people who have high blood pressure (hypertension).

Bowel problems
A low intake of dietary fiber may contribute to the development of intestinal disorders such as diverticular disease (in which small pouches form in the wall of the colon), chronic constipation, and hemorrhoids.

BALANCING YOUR DAILY DIET

One way to achieve a balanced diet is to eat a range of foods every day from the food groups described below. Sedentary adults should include at least the lower number of servings in their daily diet and more active people should aim for the higher number of servings. In addition, specific requirements for groups of people with special dietary needs are indicated where appropriate.

FOOD GROUP	SUGGESTED NUMBER OF DAILY SERVINGS
Breads, cereals, and other grain products Whole-grain and enriched varieties.	Eat six to 11 servings from the entire group and ensure that several of these servings are whole-grain products. **One serving:** One slice of bread; ½ hamburger bun or English muffin; one small roll; three to four crackers; ½ cup of cooked cereal, rice, or pasta; 1 ounce of dry cereal.
Fruits Citrus fruit, melons, berries, and all other types of fruit.	Eat three to four servings from among the items in the group. **One serving:** One piece of whole fruit such as a medium apple, banana, or orange; a grapefruit half; a melon wedge; ¾ cup of fruit juice; ½ cup of cooked or canned fruit; ¼ cup of dried fruit.
Vegetables Dark green leafy, deep yellow, and starchy vegetables, dried legumes (peas and beans), and all other types of vegetables.	Eat three to five servings from among the items in the group and use dark green leafy vegetables and cooked, dried legumes several times a week. **One serving:** ½ cup of cooked vegetables; ½ cup of chopped, raw vegetables; 1 cup of raw, leafy vegetables.
Meat, poultry, fish, and alternatives (eggs, dried beans and peas, nuts and seeds)	The daily amount should total 5 to 7 ounces of cooked lean meat, poultry, or fish. Substitute one egg, ½ cup of dried beans or peas (cooked), or 2 tablespoons of peanut butter for 1 ounce of meat or fish.
Milk, cheese, and yogurt	Have two servings. Teenagers and pregnant women require three servings or more. Teenage girls who are pregnant or breast-feeding require four servings or more. **One serving:** 1 cup of milk; 8 ounces of yogurt; 1½ ounces of natural cheese; 2 ounces of processed cheese.
Fats, sweets, and alcoholic beverages	Try to avoid consuming too much fat, sugar, and other types of sweeteners. Older people, in particular, may need to cut down on these ingredients to avoid gaining weight. If you drink alcoholic beverages, do so only in moderation and not at all during pregnancy.

BASIC WAYS TO IMPROVE YOUR DIET

You can improve your diet in the following ways:

♦ Eat as wide a variety of foods as possible.
♦ Avoid excessive consumption of all fats, especially saturated fats.
♦ Eat adequate amounts of complex carbohydrates (including whole-grain and unrefined products) and dietary fiber.
♦ Minimize intake of sugar and other sweeteners, such as syrups, honey, and molasses.
♦ Eat salt and other sodium-containing foods in moderation.
♦ Minimize your consumption of salt-cured, nitrate-processed, and smoked foods.
♦ Drink alcoholic beverages only in moderation.
♦ Increase your energy expenditure and reduce your calorie intake if you need to lose weight.
♦ Relax as you eat.

and sugar – it simply means cutting back on excess. Balance is the key. You may just need to rediscover the basics, finding new ways to prepare fresh fruits, vegetables, and other healthy foods. To assess how healthy your diet is, record what you eat for 1 or 2 weeks and compare it with the guidelines in the table above. You can use these guidelines to help plan your meals.

BALANCING A HEALTHY DIET AND A BUSY LIFE-STYLE

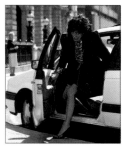

Helen Schroeder is a 38-year-old financial officer who wants to develop good eating habits and maintain a balanced diet. Because of her job, she eats out frequently. She often eats lunch on the run, and in the evenings she goes out for business or social dinners. During her personal time, she is moderately active, playing tennis twice weekly. She doesn't need to strictly limit her diet – she is not overweight, salt-sensitive, or hypertensive. We provide her with ideas for monitoring her diet to help her feel fit, stay well, and enjoy life.

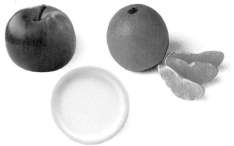

Brown-bag lunches
When you are in a hurry, it can be easy to eat an unbalanced diet that contains too many foods that are high in fat and sugar. Helen can better monitor her daytime eating if she makes her own brown-bag lunches a couple of days a week. Some simple ideas are shown below.

SANDWICHES By varying the bread and the filling, Helen can make nutritious and tasty sandwiches.

Breads
Helen can use whole-grain breads to get extra fiber. She can also select from a range of snack-size breads, such as small pita breads or rolls. Many whole-grain crackers are also nutritious and low in calories, but check labels carefully.

Fillings
Helen can choose from a wide variety of meats, fish, cheeses, and vegetables. Fillings that contain less fat include water-packed tuna, lean meat or poultry, and low-fat cottage cheese mixed with fruits or vegetables.

Additional ingredients
Condiments and spreads with little nutritional value can add fat and calorie content. Instead, Helen can choose chopped or shredded vegetables, apples, alfalfa or bean sprouts, cottage cheese, or plain low-fat yogurt.

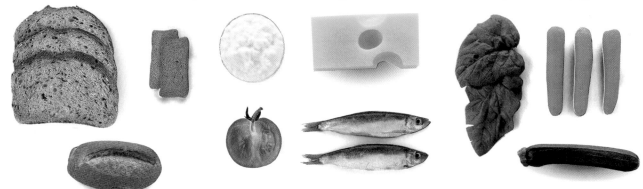

SALADS
Helen can create imaginative salads by combining ingredients such as raw or cooked vegetables, cheese, cooked dried beans, whole-grain pasta, and brown rice. Low-fat dressing, yogurt, tofu, or blended cottage cheese are tasty low-calorie toppings.

HOT LUNCHES
For a change, Helen can take soup or a casserole to reheat in the office microwave. Soups can be prepared quickly using frozen vegetables and dried herbs. Helen doesn't drink milk regularly so milk-based soups are a good choice as a source of calcium. She can use low-fat milk or powdered milk to reduce the fat content.

SNACKS AND DESSERTS
Fresh fruits are always a nutritious addition to a brown-bag lunch and are a handy snack. Yogurt with fresh fruit also makes a low-fat, healthy dessert or snack. Helen doesn't need to eliminate sweets altogether but she should eat them in moderate amounts and balance them with other foods that are lower in fat, sugar, and calories.

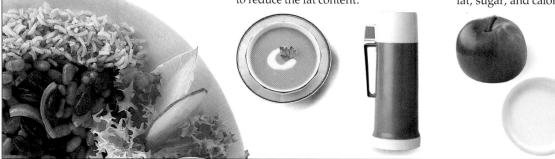

EATING OUT AT RESTAURANTS

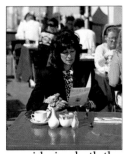

Helen enjoys eating at restaurants. She wants guidelines for choosing meals that are part of a balanced diet and are not too high in fats, calories, or sugar. Many restaurants now adjust their cooking to suit health-conscious people. Helen should study the menu before making a selection, considering both the preparation and ingredients. For example, grilled and broiled foods tend to be lower in fat than deep-fried foods. The terms poached, steamed, stir-fried, and roasted also usually signal a lower fat content. Helen doesn't need to cut out all her favorite foods. If she splurges on one course, she can cut back on others. She can also adjust her diet the next day to balance her fat intake. Some diners need to watch their salt intake more carefully because conditions such as hypertension make them salt-sensitive. It may be difficult to identify foods with a lower sodium content, but condiments such as soy sauce are almost always high in sodium.

MENU

APPETIZERS

Fresh melon

Fried wonton (F) (S) (Na)
Served with sweet and sour sauce

Fresh fruit medley
Served in a pineapple boat

Chicken liver pâté (F) (Na)
Served with melba toast

Gazpacho
A crunchy soup of blended tomatoes, cucumbers, garlic, green pepper, and onion, served chilled

Shrimp cocktail
Served with a spicy cocktail sauce on the side

ENTRÉES

Baked chicken breast
Boneless breast of chicken baked in a delicate lemon basil sauce

Southern-style chicken (F) (Na)
Fried to a crispy, golden brown

Beef en brochette
Skewered cubes of beef with fresh mushroom caps

Barbecued baby back ribs (F) (S) (Na)
A hefty rack of broiled pork ribs smothered with hickory-smoked barbecue sauce

Veal tenderloin (F) (S) (Na)
Plump medallions of veal in a rich cream sauce with mushrooms and capers

Fish and chips (F) (Na)
Fresh filet of sole dipped in a special beer batter and deep-fried, served with french-fried potatoes

VEGETABLES

French-fried potatoes (F)

Herbed new potatoes

Creamy coleslaw (F) (S)

Steamed zucchini-carrot medley

Garden fresh peas with pearl onions

DESSERTS

Fresh fruit sorbet
Assorted flavors

Poached pears
With raspberry glaze

Assorted fresh pastries (F) (S)
Rich, flaky pastries with assorted fillings

Apple dumpling (F) (S)
Whole apple baked in a flaky cinnamon pastry, topped with whipped cream and chopped pecans

Ice cream sundae (F) (S)
A rich French vanilla, topped with fudge sauce, nuts, and whipped cream, served with a cookie

Fresh strawberries (in season)

KEY	
These items are higher in:	
(F)	Fats
(S)	Sugar
(Na)	Sodium

Making balanced choices
The codes on the menu indicate dishes that are higher in fats, sugar, and sodium (see key). The other dishes are lower in all these components and generally contain fewer calories.

TIPS FOR EATING OUT

♦ Ask about serving sizes. Are half portions available?
♦ Choose an appetizer as a main dish, share a dish, or have an appetizer and a salad.
♦ Ask about preparation and ingredients. Is butter or other fat used for broiling? Are vegetables served with butter?
♦ Ask if fish, chicken, or meat can be broiled without added fat. Ask if chicken can be prepared without the skin.
♦ Ask to have any sauces or dressings served on the side.
♦ Ask for foods not listed on the menu, such as low-fat or skim milk, fresh fruit, or plain yogurt.

YOUR GENERAL HEALTH

YOUR GENERAL HEALTH reflects the condition of each of your body parts and systems. While each part or system can be considered individually, it is important to remember that your body functions as an integrated whole. If one part of your body starts to malfunction, your overall sense of well-being will be diminished. To monitor your health, you need to be alert to changes in each of the systems and parts of your body. These pages illustrate the complexity of the human body and its components.

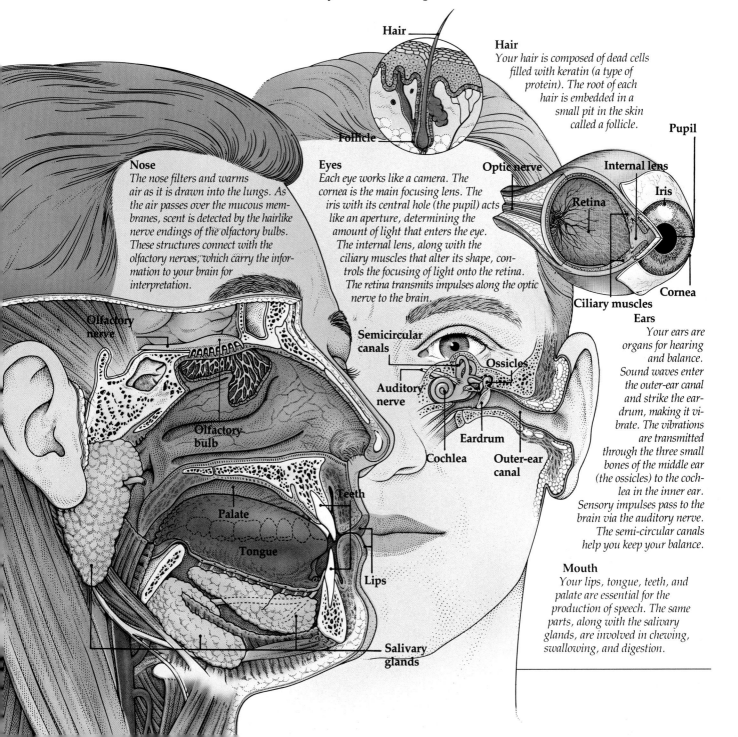

Hair

Hair
Your hair is composed of dead cells filled with keratin (a type of protein). The root of each hair is embedded in a small pit in the skin called a follicle.

Follicle

Nose
The nose filters and warms air as it is drawn into the lungs. As the air passes over the mucous membranes, scent is detected by the hairlike nerve endings of the olfactory bulbs. These structures connect with the olfactory nerves, which carry the information to your brain for interpretation.

Eyes
Each eye works like a camera. The cornea is the main focusing lens. The iris with its central hole (the pupil) acts like an aperture, determining the amount of light that enters the eye. The internal lens, along with the ciliary muscles that alter its shape, controls the focusing of light onto the retina. The retina transmits impulses along the optic nerve to the brain.

Optic nerve

Pupil

Internal lens

Iris

Retina

Cornea

Ciliary muscles

Olfactory nerve

Olfactory bulb

Semicircular canals

Auditory nerve

Ossicles

Eardrum

Cochlea

Outer-ear canal

Ears
Your ears are organs for hearing and balance. Sound waves enter the outer-ear canal and strike the eardrum, making it vibrate. The vibrations are transmitted through the three small bones of the middle ear (the ossicles) to the cochlea in the inner ear. Sensory impulses pass to the brain via the auditory nerve. The semi-circular canals help you keep your balance.

Palate

Tongue

Teeth

Lips

Salivary glands

Mouth
Your lips, tongue, teeth, and palate are essential for the production of speech. The same parts, along with the salivary glands, are involved in chewing, swallowing, and digestion.

Hands
Your hands are the most flexible parts of your skeleton, enabling you to hold and manipulate objects. The forearm muscles, connected via tendons to the bones in your hand, control most movement. Short muscles in your palm control other actions.

Muscles

Tendons

Tendons connected to forearm muscles

Ligaments

Bones

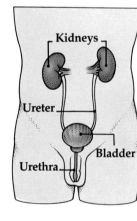

Urinary tract
The kidneys form urine by filtering blood. The urine passes down the ureters and collects in the bladder. Pressure on the muscles of the bladder triggers the urge to urinate; the urine is passed through the urethra.

Kidneys

Ureter

Urethra

Bladder

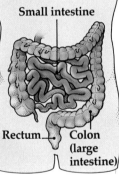

Intestines
The small intestine digests food and absorbs nutrients into the bloodstream. In the large intestine (the colon), water from the undigested material is absorbed and the residue (feces) passes into the rectum for excretion.

Small intestine

Rectum

Colon (large intestine)

Feet
Each foot is made up of 26 bones, 19 muscles, and more than 100 ligaments and tendons. Your feet are strong and flexible to support your weight and propel you forward when you walk.

Skin
Your skin has two layers. The epidermis, the outer protective layer, has a covering of dead cells. The dermis underneath contains most of the living structures. Underneath the dermis and over the muscles is a fatty layer of tissue.

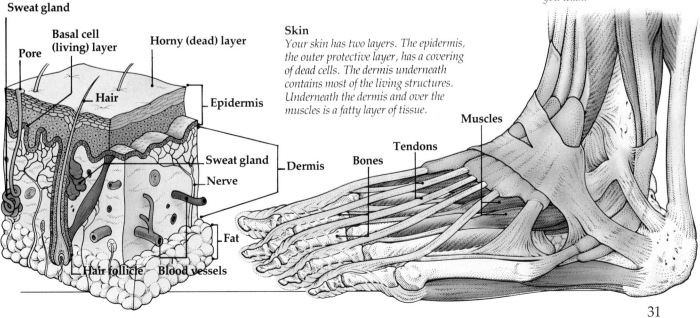

Sweat gland

Pore

Basal cell (living) layer

Hair

Horny (dead) layer

Epidermis

Sweat gland

Dermis

Nerve

Fat

Hair follicle

Blood vessels

Bones

Tendons

Muscles

31

HOW IS YOUR VISION?

Your vision can change in several ways. The most common problems involve errors of refraction, the mechanism by which an image is focused on the retina. These errors affect your visual acuity (the sharpness of your vision). Corrective lenses can almost always resolve the blurriness caused by a refractive error. Other types of defective vision may be the result of disorders of the eye or optic nerve or of the nerve pathways to the brain. These vision disorders may cause altered visual acuity or interference with your field of vision. Corrective lenses will not eliminate these problems.

If you notice any persistent change in the quality of your vision, report it promptly to your doctor. Further medical evaluation is needed.

Focusing problems

Problems of focusing (refractive errors) usually occur either because of defects present at birth or because of the natural aging process. Some people are born with nearsightedness (the inability to focus at long distances), farsightedness

---

EFFECT OF AGE ON VISION

A younger person is able to focus his or her eyes easily on objects at widely differing distances because the internal lenses of the eyes have a natural elasticity that allows the curvature of the lenses to change. The eye lenses gradually and progressively become less elastic with age, and accommodation power weakens. As a result, the nearest point on which the eye can focus moves farther away. Even if your vision has always been normal, you may require reading glasses after about age 45.

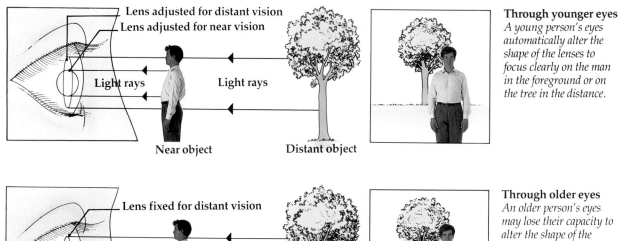

Through younger eyes
A young person's eyes automatically alter the shape of the lenses to focus clearly on the man in the foreground or on the tree in the distance.

Through older eyes
An older person's eyes may lose their capacity to alter the shape of the lenses, thus hindering the ability to focus clearly on the man in the foreground. The lenses become fixed at a focus for distant objects.

CAN YOU READ THIS?
As close focusing power decreases, the smallest print that you can see at reading distance must be larger. Hold this book 16 inches away and look at the print at right (wearing any corrective lenses you need for distance vision). Your ability to read the print is a crude indication of your close focusing power. People under 45 can often read even the smallest size. People over 65 may have difficulty reading the largest.

Can you read this?

Can you read this?

Can you read this?

(the inability to focus at short distances), and/or astigmatism (an uneven curvature of the transparent front portion of the eye, the cornea, which distorts vision). Problems of accommodation – your eyes' automatic ability to focus on near objects – develop with age. This type of defect is usually helped by wearing bifocal lenses.

CHECK YOUR VISION

Check your vision by answering the questions below. Check each eye separately, covering the other eye completely. If any answer indicates that you have problems with vision, discuss them with your doctor. Many problems can be corrected with glasses or contact lenses. However, if you have an eye disease, prompt treatment is vital.

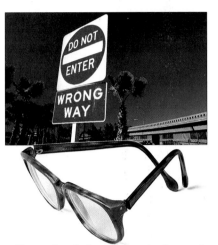

♦ **When you look at objects in the distance, such as street signs, do they appear blurred?** If so, you may need correction for your near-sightedness.

♦ **Can you read fairly small print at 16 inches?** If not, you may need reading glasses or contact lenses to correct farsightedness.

♦ **If you already have corrective lenses for distance vision, do distant objects appear blurred when you are wearing your glasses or contact lenses?** If so, you may need a stronger prescription.

♦ **If your near vision is blurred when you are wearing your reading glasses, does the image become clear when you move the print farther away?** If so, you need a stronger prescription.

♦ **Is any part of your field of vision blurred or absent?** If so, you may have an eye disease. Seek treatment promptly.

♦ **Do you bump into objects on either side of you?** If so, have your visual field checked. You can also try the test on this page.

Do you have astigmatism?
Look at the pattern below. Are all the lines clearly focused? If only some are clear, your cornea may not be truly spherical (although your eye is healthy) and you probably have astigmatism. Astigmatism can be corrected with glasses or contact lenses.

Test your visual field
This test checks whether you have an abnormally restricted field of vision. Look directly ahead at a fixed object and cover one eye with your hand. Stretch your other hand out to the side at shoulder level with your thumb pointing up. Wiggle your thumb. You should be able to detect the movement without altering your gaze. Test the other eye. If you have to move your hand about a foot forward to detect your thumb moving, you may have a problem with peripheral vision.

Diseases of the eye

Some diseases can cause changes in the transparency of the parts of the eye through which light passes – the cornea, lens, and vitreous humor (a jellylike substance inside the eye). Other disorders, such as diabetes, can lead to defects in the retina or optic nerve at the back of the eye. Some diseases are more common in old age. Cataract, a gradual loss of transparency of the lens, usually occurs later in life. Its cause is not known. Glaucoma, which is abnormally high pressure of the fluid of the eye, rarely occurs before age 40 and often causes no symptoms until the advanced stages. Macular degeneration of the retina causes a roughly circular area of blindness in the center of the visual field. Problems such as these require evaluation by an ophthalmologist. Sometimes the effects of these diseases are permanent, but early treatment may help preserve vision.

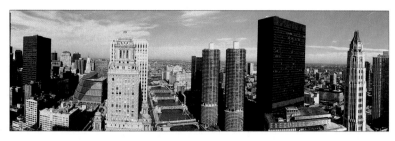

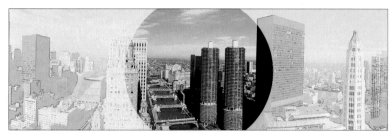

Tunnel vision
A progressive decrease in your ability to detect objects that are not directly in front of you may mean that your eye is being damaged by a disease such as glaucoma. In this condition the pressure inside the eyes is excessive. Untreated glaucoma can cause permanent damage to internal blood vessels and/or optic nerve fibers.

Black curtain

Halos around lights

Scattering of light

Spots before the eyes

WARNING

If you see halos around lights or spots before your eyes, experience mistiness or cloudiness of vision or changes in your perception of color, or if you see sudden flashes of light, scattering of light, or a black curtain coming across your field of vision, you may have an eye disease. Seek professional treatment immediately.

Sudden flashes of light

Cloudiness of vision

PROFESSIONAL VISION CHECKUP

If you have problems with your vision you should have a professional eye checkup every 2 years. If you have diabetes or high blood pressure, have your eyes examined at least once a year. Even if you have good vision you should begin to have regular checkups after the age of 40.

Your family doctor can check your distance vision using the Snellen's chart and your accommodation power (ability to focus on near objects) using a near-vision chart bearing print of different sizes. If these tests suggest a problem, you will be referred to an ophthalmologist. He or she will repeat the test with the Snellen's chart, placing different lenses in front of your eyes to calculate the type of glasses or contact lenses you may need. If your vision is not corrected by these lenses, you may have an eye disease that requires more tests and treatment.

During an eye examination, the ophthalmologist will also examine the inside of your eyes with an ophthalmoscope to look for any changes caused by disease. If you are over 40, he or she will measure the pressure of the fluid inside your eyes to check for glaucoma. Your field of vision should also be checked. Regular periodic examinations such as these are the best way to ensure that the effects of advancing age are detected and treated to preserve your vision as much as possible.

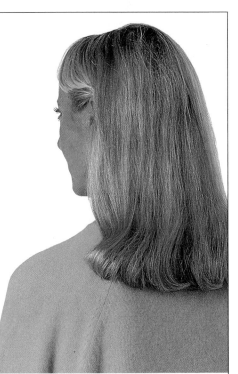

Snellen's chart
Visual acuity (the sharpness of your vision) is tested with the Snellen's chart at 20 feet. The eyes are tested one at a time, with and without any lenses you wear to correct distance vision.

Color vision test
The most common defect of color vision is difficulty distinguishing between reds and greens. Test each of your eyes separately for red-green color vision by looking at the Ishihara's test plate reproduced on the left. You should be able to see the figure 8. People who have difficulty distinguishing between red and green will see the figure 3. Your doctor can give you a more precise color vision test.

Retinoscopy
A retinoscope is used to determine the degree of a refractive error – nearsightedness, farsightedness, or astigmatism. A narrow beam of light is projected into your eye from the retinoscope. The doctor makes small movements of the light source and observes the movement of the beam reflected back through your pupil.

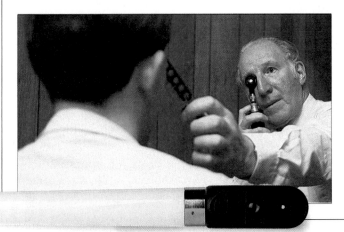

Visual field test
The doctor may use an instrument such as that shown to make an accurate test of your visual field. One eye is covered. With the other eye you look straight ahead at a fixed point. Points of light then appear at different positions on the screen and your perception of each point is diagrammed.

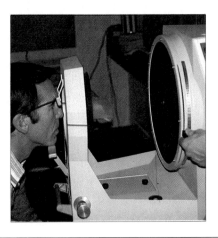

HOW IS YOUR HEARING?

You can experience two general categories of hearing loss. Conductive loss is the result of faulty conduction of sound from the outside to the inner ear via the eardrum and the ossicles, the tiny bones of the middle ear. The other type of hearing loss, sensorineural loss, is caused by a failure of the eighth cranial nerve, the nerve of hearing, or of the cochlea. The cochlea converts the mechanical vibration of the eardrum and ossicles to neural impulses. Sensorineural hearing loss is usually not reversible. However, it can almost always be helped by use of a hearing aid, which increases the volume of the sounds entering the ear.

Sensorineural hearing loss

Sensorineural hearing loss usually affects detection of the higher tones that form hissing sounds. It may make it difficult to understand speech. Many of us experience a degree of sensorineural hearing loss as we get older. However, this loss can be made worse by exposure to loud noises. Sensorineural hearing loss may also be caused by some poisons or drugs. High doses of aspirin or some diuretics may cause a temporary hearing loss. Certain antibiotics (and at least one

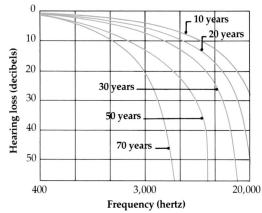

Hearing loss with age
As you get older, your sensitivity to high-frequency sounds is reduced, so that the higher pitched a sound is, the louder it must be for you to hear it. Aging may also affect your sensitivity to lower tones and may interfere with your ability to distinguish individual words in conversation.

CHECK YOUR HEARING

You can check your hearing by answering the questions and performing the tests shown below. While fairly rudimentary, these tests offer a useful idea of the severity of a hearing problem and of the difference between your ears. (Test each ear separately, while blocking sound as completely as possible from the other ear.) If you seriously suspect that you may have a hearing loss, seek the advice of your doctor. He or she may refer you to an otolaryngologist, a doctor who specializes in disorders of the head and neck.

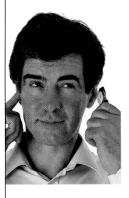

1 See if you can hear the tick of a windup watch.

2 Rub your finger and thumb together at varying distances from your ear, and note when you stop hearing the sound. Compare your responses to those of someone with good hearing.

♦ **Do you find conversation difficult to follow in noisy surroundings?** If so, you may have a minor defect of hearing.

♦ **Do you find conversation difficult to follow in quiet surroundings?** If so, you may have a major defect of hearing.

♦ **Do you hear the top four notes on a piano as having definite, pitched sounds?** If not, you have a hearing loss in the high tones – a feature of sensorineural hearing loss.

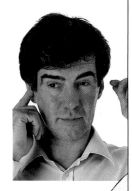

anticancer drug) may cause permanent hearing loss. If you think you may have a sensorineural hearing loss, do not hesitate to consult your doctor.

Conductive hearing loss

Conductive hearing loss may be caused by wax (cerumen) in the ear canal or by fluid in the normally air-filled middle ear. This fluid is usually a temporary effect of an upper respiratory tract infection. Malfunction of the ossicles also causes a conductive loss as the result of a congenital abnormality, infection, aging, or otosclerosis (a hereditary progressive disorder of the ossicles that usually begins in early adulthood).

WARNING

Consult your doctor if you have any of these symptoms after a cold or a throat infection:

♦ Severe earache and fever
♦ Full feeling in ear and hearing loss
♦ Continuing difficulty hearing conversation
♦ Ringing or buzzing in ear

COULD YOU BENEFIT FROM A HEARING AID?

Hearing aids are probably the most important component of modern hearing rehabilitation. No one needs to feel self-conscious about wearing these devices anymore because they have become far less obvious and more convenient for the user over the years. The first hearing aids had a microphone, battery, and electronics in a small box that the user carried in his or her pocket. Later models were developed to attach to glasses or to be worn behind the ear. Today, most people wear devices that fit entirely inside the outer ear or the ear canal (see illustration at right). In the future, surgically implantable hearing aids may become more widespread. In addition to the miniaturization of the device, advances in electronics have brought improved performance. Today, your doctor can closely match the amplification to your hearing loss. For instance, if you have a high-tone loss, you can be fitted with a hearing aid that amplifies only the high tones and not the low ones. As technology advances, hearing aids will be developed that will more effectively limit unwanted sounds so that the user can hear better in noisy environments.

Today's hearing aid

ARE YOU BEING EXPOSED TO DAMAGING NOISE?

The volume of sound is measured on a decibel (dB) scale. Your hearing may be injured if subjected to sounds over 80 decibels for an extended period of time. Hearing is likely to be damaged by even brief exposure to sounds over 110 decibels. Use ear protection during any noisy activities. Noise may be damaging your ears if you experience any of the following:

♦ Persistent ringing in your ears after exposure to noise
♦ Any hearing loss, however brief, after exposure to noise
♦ Any pain associated with the noise

Motorcycle at 25 feet
90 decibels

Chain saw at 3 feet
110 decibels

Pneumatic drill at 3 feet
120 decibels

PROFESSIONAL HEARING CHECKUP

In some hearing tests, a vibrating tuning fork is placed on your forehead or on the bone behind your ear to test bone conduction; it is placed near your outer-ear canal to test air conduction. For tests to measure your hearing, a machine called an audiometer transmits sounds of different frequencies and loudness to each ear while the other ear is covered completely. The volume of each sound is progressively decreased, and you are asked to indicate when you can no longer hear the sound. The results are recorded on a chart called an audiogram.

Normal audiogram
When hearing is normal, sounds of 25 decibels or lower are audible across the range of frequencies by both air conduction (circles) and bone conduction (arrows).

Abnormal audiogram
With conductive hearing loss, air conduction hearing levels (circles) are diminished, but bone conduction hearing levels (arrows) are normal.

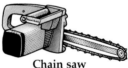

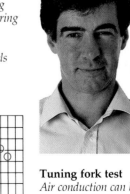

Tuning fork test
Air conduction can be tested by holding a vibrating tuning fork near the opening of the ear canal.

MONITORING YOUR ORAL HEALTH

You have good reason to regularly check inside your mouth. First, you can easily see signs of gingivitis, which is gum disease at an early, reversible stage. Mild gingivitis is common among young adults who do not floss. Second, many mouth diseases produce obvious (and sometimes painful) changes. Early detection is critical, especially with oral cancer. Third, some mouth conditions are symptoms of a more widespread disease (see below). In addition to performing oral inspections at home, you should have a professional dental examination at least once a year. Have one more frequently if your dentist recommends it.

EXAMINING YOUR MOUTH

Regularly examine your lips, gums, teeth, tongue, and mouth lining in front of a mirror in a good light. Remove any dental prosthesis before you begin. The signs of a healthy mouth are described in the list below. Some potential problems are illustrated at the bottom of the page. Consult your dentist if you discover anything odd or have a recurrent oral problem. You should also see your dentist if any of your teeth become sensitive to hot and cold or if you have a persistent or recurrent toothache.

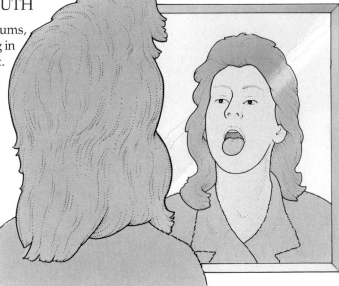

WARNING SIGNS OF ORAL CANCER

Cancer can affect any of the tissues in your mouth. Smokers (including cigar and pipe smokers), tobacco chewers, and heavy drinkers should be particularly alert to the warning signs. Consult your doctor or dentist if you notice any of the following:

♦ A sore on your lips, gums, or mouth lining that does not heal within 2 to 3 weeks
♦ Any white patch inside your mouth or on your lips
♦ Any swelling or lump inside your mouth or on your lips or tongue, whether or not it is painful and whether or not it is spreading
♦ Numbness or pain in your mouth or throat with no apparent cause
♦ Repeated bleeding in your mouth with no apparent cause

CHECKLIST FOR A HEALTHY MOUTH

♦ Firm, pink gums with well-defined edges
♦ Some areas of dark pigmentation, depending on your racial group
♦ Smooth, glistening, reddish-pink mouth-lining surfaces

♦ Well-concealed tooth roots
♦ Off-white or yellowish teeth, free from stains, deposits, or cavities
♦ A rough-surfaced tongue of an even color, occasionally with small fissures

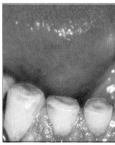

Bleeding gums
Redness, swelling, and bleeding of the gums are signs of gum disease. Gingivitis, the earliest stage of gum disease, can usually be reversed with better oral hygiene, including daily flossing.

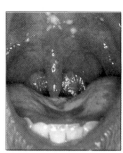

Abnormal wear
Fine cracks and worn areas in the teeth are normal with aging, but severe wear and loss of tooth height may be a sign of unconscious biting and grinding known as bruxism.

Mouth infections
An infection, such as the fungal infection candidiasis (white patches shown here), may affect the mouth lining or tongue. Your doctor should investigate any signs of oral infection.

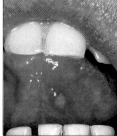

Mouth ulcers
Painful mouth ulcers may occur singly or in clusters. Some women experience mouth ulcers during the course of their menstrual cycles. Iron deficiency can also sometimes be the cause.

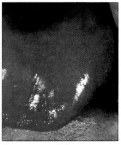

Soreness of the tongue
A sore, bright red, unnaturally smooth tongue, such as the one shown above, can be a sign of anemia or of a vitamin deficiency and requires medical investigation.

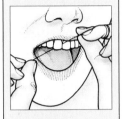

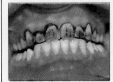
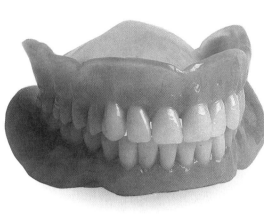

Checking the fit of your dentures
Changes in your gums and the bone that supports them may require you to replace your dentures periodically. Badly fitting dentures can cause serious problems, so have your dentures checked during your regular dental examination. Consult your dentist if your dentures become loose or uncomfortable in any way.

PROFESSIONAL DENTAL CHECKUP

During a checkup, the dentist examines the surfaces of the mouth tissue, the lips, the tongue, the gums, and the teeth for signs of disease. The dentist also looks for signs of an abnormal bite or of clenching and grinding of the teeth (bruxism). He or she also assesses the effectiveness of your oral hygiene. If you wear dentures, their fit and function will be evaluated. Finally, your teeth may be scaled to remove hard, crustlike deposits of calculus (tartar); they are then polished and flossed.

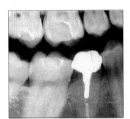

Dental X-rays
Your dentist may take X-rays periodically to reveal decay and to detect any bone loss from periodontitis (gum disease). The white areas show dental work.

HOW WELL CAN YOU SMELL AND TASTE?

Taste and smell are vital to the enjoyment of food, and they also can warn you of danger. Your sense of taste depends largely on food odors that pass through the back of the throat into the nose. The taste buds on your tongue can detect only basic sensations. The delicate hairlike fronds at the upper, inner ends of the nasal passage can recognize tens of thousands of different odors. Taste and smell become less acute with age. Allergies, nasal polyps, recurrent infections, and some medications may also decrease the taste/smell sensations. The fragile organs for smell are easily damaged by air polluted with tobacco smoke or industrial poisons.

Testing taste
Using four cotton swabs, apply sugar, lemon juice, salt, and quinine (tonic) water to the tongue of the person being tested. Ask the person to identify the flavor by pointing to the written word (sweet, sour, salty, or bitter). Test one side of the tongue at a time. The mouth should be rinsed with water after each flavor.

Testing your sense of smell
Select a variety of aromatic, nonirritating substances, such as soap, coffee, lemon peel, a peeled clove of garlic, and a stick of cinnamon. Blindfold the person to be tested and place each odor-releasing substance below one nostril. Test each nostril separately by blocking the other one.

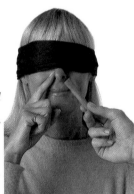

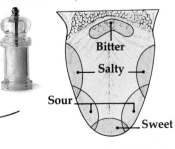

Taste areas
Different areas of the tongue seem to be more sensitive to each of the four basic tastes.

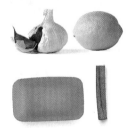

LOOK IN THE MIRROR– IS YOUR FACE HEALTHY?

Your face can reveal more important facts about your health or the presence of different diseases than almost any other part of your body. It can reflect an underlying general disease, deficiencies in your nutritional state, and the effects of emotional stress, aging, skin disorders, allergic reactions, and damaging habits such as tobacco smoking or excessive alcohol consumption.

Change in color or shape

Changes to watch for include those that affect facial coloring, including the lips and the whites of the eyes. Any redness, yellowing, blue tinge, unusual paleness, or darkening should be noted. Alterations in the shape or size of your face may also indicate a health problem. Your face may become fatter or thinner, or features such as your bones or eyes may become more or less prominent.

A yellow tinge
A yellow tinge to your skin and the whites of your eyes may mean you have jaundice as a result of liver disease (shown right). Jaundice also is sometimes caused by anemia, which destroys the red blood cells.

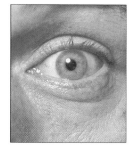

Malar flush
Increased color over your cheekbones may indicate that the mitral valve of your heart has narrowed. However, this coloring does not necessarily mean you have heart disease.

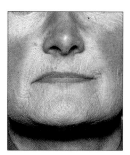

Lupus erythematosus
This photograph shows the characteristic butterfly-shaped rash of lupus erythematosus, which can become a serious inflammatory condition that affects the body's connective tissues.

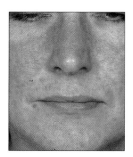

FACIAL COLOR
Pallor (paleness) is one of the most common changes in skin color. It may indicate anemia caused by iron deficiency, blood loss, or other conditions. Under emergency circumstances, pallor may also indicate that a person is in shock. A bluish hue to the lips – cyanosis – can indicate a serious lung or heart condition. Patches of depigmented skin may indicate vitiligo, a disorder caused by absence of the cells that secrete the skin pigment melanin. Some other typical changes in facial color are illustrated on this page.

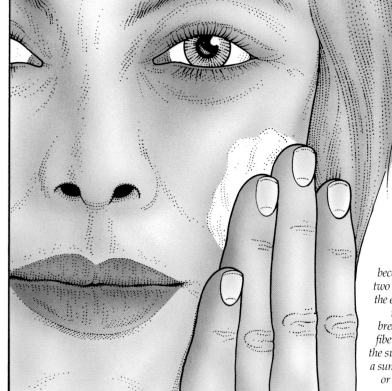

Can you reverse sun damage?
In recent years, widespread publicity has focused on use of retinoid creams to reverse the damaging effects of the sun. Retinoids can correct only small, fine wrinkles and not large, deep ones. Long-term studies are being done to determine if significant benefits will be gained.

You can minimize sun exposure
Your skin, especially sun-exposed areas like your face, becomes less elastic with age for two main reasons – heredity and the effects of the sun's rays. These rays penetrate your skin and break down collagen and elastic fibers. Control your exposure to the sun by using a sun block with a sun protection factor (SPF) of 15 or higher every day and wear a hat and sunglasses.

FLUSHING OR RASHES
Some people normally flush after consuming alcohol or a spicy food or if they are in a hot environment. If it is persistent, flushing may be due to rosacea – a skin disorder of unknown cause. A facial rash that appears after exposure to sunlight may be a reaction to medications such as sulfa drugs, tetracycline drugs, or barbiturates.

Facial skin conditions

Some skin disorders affect the face in particular. These include acne and certain rashes, allergies, and infections. Some skin problems reflect your general health. For example, if you have a cold, cold sores may appear around the mouth area, caused by infection with the virus that causes herpes simplex. Eczema is often worsened by stress, and the appearance of acne may coincide with menstruation. Other kinds of mild dermatitis (literally, inflammation of the skin) also commonly occur on the face. Your doctor can help distinguish one kind from another and provide effective treatment. Skin cancers most commonly occur on the face. They are almost 100 percent curable.

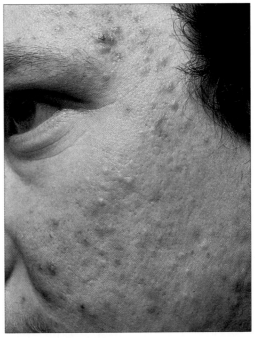

Acne
Pimples, whiteheads, and blackheads on the cheeks, chin, and forehead are characteristic of acne. Effective treatment is now available for this condition. Early treatment is important, especially to prevent permanent scarring. Acne sometimes develops in adulthood. A woman's acne often gets worse before or during her menstrual period; this type of acne is related to hormonal changes. If you are being treated for acne, remember that your skin takes more than a month to regenerate, so you may have to wait 4 to 8 weeks to see an improvement.

YOUR HAIR AND SCALP

On the average, we lose 100 to 150 (out of a total of 300,000) scalp hairs each day. This hair is usually replaced by new hair growing in underneath. Hair growth in both men and women responds to hormonal changes. Among women, hair growth may alter during pregnancy, childbirth, and menopause.

If you find you are losing hair excessively and persistently, it may be a sign of an underlying medical disorder. Sudden loss of hair, resulting in patches of

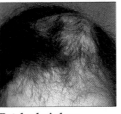

Patchy hair loss
The most common type of patchy hair loss on the scalp is alopecia areata. Its cause is not known. Round, bald patches appear and the exposed scalp looks healthy.

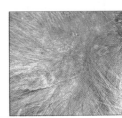

Fungal infections
Fungal scalp infections such as ringworm may also produce hair loss in patches. These patches are characterized by reddened, ring-shaped, scaly areas on the scalp.

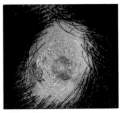

Skin disorders affecting the scalp
Some skin disorders interfere with hair growth. The photograph shows lichen planus, an inflammatory skin disease.

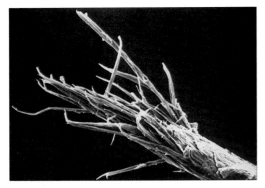

Split ends
This color-enhanced photograph shows a scalp hair with a split end (magnification ×125). Excessive shampooing, combing, or blow-drying your hair using a high heat setting cracks the hair cuticle (the outer cell layer) and makes hair more likely to split.

Male pattern baldness
The most common form of hair loss, male pattern baldness, is an inherited trait. The pattern of loss starts at the temples and the crown and gradually widens. Some regrowth of hair has occurred in some balding men undergoing treatment with minoxidil, an agent that elongates follicles in bald areas. Minoxidil does not cause new follicles to form.

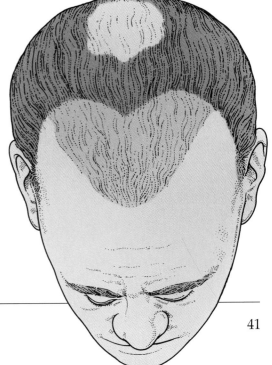

41

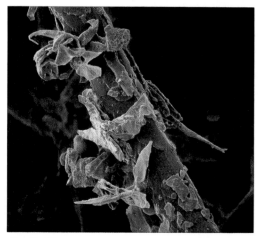

Dandruff
Dandruff, shown coating a strand of hair in the photograph above (magnification ×1,000), is the abnormal accumulation of small flakes of dead skin on the scalp. It poses no health risk but is commonly associated with mild seborrheic dermatitis, which causes an itchy rash.

baldness, is usually caused by skin disorders that affect the scalp or by scalp infections. By contrast, a gradual, overall hair loss sometimes happens 3 to 6 months after a feverish illness, severe shock, an accident, pregnancy, or surgery. Treatment with some drugs (such as anticancer drugs) may cause widespread hair loss as well.

MONITORING SKIN CHANGES

Many skin changes occur as part of the natural aging process. Your life-style and habits, such as smoking, drinking alcohol, or exposure to the sun, can accelerate these age-related effects. It is important to be able to identify any abnormal changes in your skin that may indicate a health problem. Changes can be caused by skin disorders or may be manifestations of a general disease involving other body systems. A purple skin rash that accompanies a sudden illness may be caused by septicemia (blood poisoning from a bacterial infection). Any skin blemish that changes in appearance or becomes itchy or painful should be checked by your doctor to ensure that it is not skin cancer (see SKIN SELF-EXAMINATION on page 54).

(see SKIN SELF-EXAMINATION on page 54).

HAIR ANALYSIS
Hair (or nail clippings) contains material that can provide a record of the chemical makeup of the body in recent months and even in recent years if the hair is long enough. Analysis of hair can detect the presence or absence of drugs such as cocaine or morphine, providing clear-cut evidence of drug abuse or of abstention from drugs. However, the claims of any clinics that maintain hair analysis enables them to detect deficiencies of vitamins and trace elements are unproven.

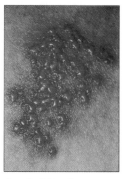

A painful rash
A painful rash can be caused by shingles, an infection of the nerves supplying the skin. The infection is brought on by the herpesvirus (the same virus that causes chickenpox). The virus may lie dormant for years before emerging when resistance to disease is low.

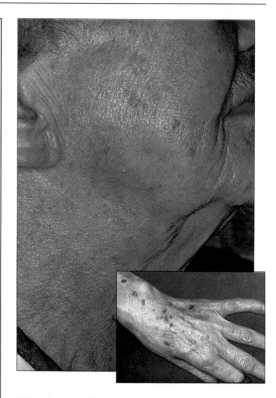

Skin changes that occur with age
In addition to loss of skin elasticity with age, patchy darkening of the skin often develops (age spots). Purple-brown spots or patches (known as senile purpura) are also common, especially among middle-aged or older women. They are caused by fragile blood vessels bleeding under the skin. These normal changes should be distinguished from the discoloration that occurs as a result of a disorder. If you have any doubt about the cause of skin changes, consult your doctor.

YOUR HANDS

Your hands can provide helpful information about your state of health. They contain parts of many of your body systems, including your skin, bones, joints, muscles, connective tissues, tendons, blood vessels, and nerves, each of which can be affected by a variety of general diseases or infections. Problems caused by environmental factors may also be apparent. Any alteration in the appearance of your hands and nails, unusual sensations, and any restriction of hand movements may indicate a variety of generalized conditions such as certain forms of arthritis, some types of anemia, or disorders related to certain types of occupational hazards.

WHAT YOUR HANDS MAY REVEAL

If you notice any unusual changes in the characteristics of your hands, such as the ones described below, discuss them with your doctor.

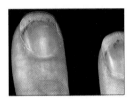

Splinter hemorrhages
Splinter-shaped blood blisters under your nails can result from injury; it is normal to have one or two of these blisters at a time. If there are many, they may indicate infective endocarditis, a serious heart disorder.

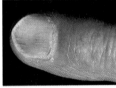

Flattened, spoon-shaped, brittle nails
These may indicate that you are deficient in iron.

HAND TREMORS

A hand tremor while the hand is at rest and slowness of movement when touching each finger to thumb in turn may indicate you have Parkinson's disease, a brain disorder that affects movement. In contrast, a general feeling of shakiness and hand trembling that occurs when you are trying to write or perform tasks that require delicate finger movements may mean you are anxious or that you have an overactive thyroid gland.

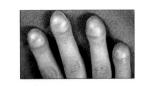

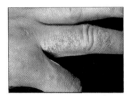

Clubbing of the fingers
Excessively rounded nails may indicate one of several serious diseases of the heart, lungs, liver, or intestines.

Itchy redness
Redness, cracking, scaling, and itching of the skin may be eczema. Contact with substances such as paint remover, or with materials you are allergic to, can also cause a rash.

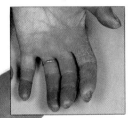

Raynaud's phenomenon
Fingers that turn white and then blue on exposure to cold may indicate that you have Raynaud's phenomenon, in which there is instability in the caliber of the blood vessels to the extremities.

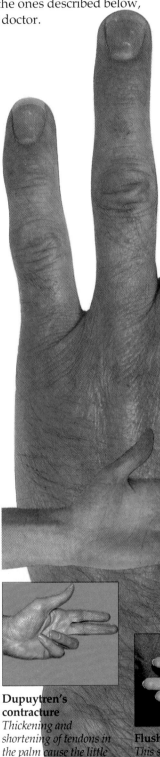

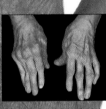

Rheumatoid arthritis
Swollen, tender, and painful wrist, knuckle, or finger joints and difficulty forming a fist may mean you have rheumatoid arthritis.

TINGLING AND NUMBNESS

A tingling and numbness in your thumb and fingers (and sometimes your whole palm) that tends to be worse at night may mean you have carpal tunnel syndrome. In this condition, swollen tissues in the wrist joint cause pressure on the nerve running through it, leading to some nerve damage.

Dupuytren's contracture
Thickening and shortening of tendons in the palm cause the little finger and other fingers to become permanently bent. This condition can be corrected by a minor operation.

Flushed palms
This sign may confirm a diagnosis of liver disease, providing other signs are present. Palms may also be reddened for no detectable reason.

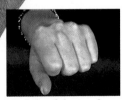

Nodule of the tendon
A lumpy nodule on the back of your hand may be a fatty deposit. It occurs in people with hyperlipidemia, an inherited disorder in which the level of fats in the blood is abnormally high.

SWEATING

The average person has about 3 million sweat glands. Sweat production varies widely among individuals, and it may occur under many different circumstances. For example, while sweating is mainly the process by which the body cools itself, it also is a response to fear or psychological stress. It is more profuse in teenagers and young adults, in women approaching the menopause, and in those who are overweight. You may perspire more after eating hot or spicy foods, after drinking alcohol, or after taking aspirin. Excessive sweating is a normal response to a fever. Perhaps the most common cause of increased sweating is the wearing of clothes made of synthetic fibers. The fibers do not absorb moisture or allow sweat to evaporate.

BODY ODOR
The sweat produced by the glands in the armpits always carries an aroma, which varies from person to person. The sweat from other parts of the body has no smell unless it remains on the skin or in clothes. Bacteria acting on the perspiration may then produce an unpleasant smell that can be avoided simply by bathing and changing clothing, especially underclothes, daily.

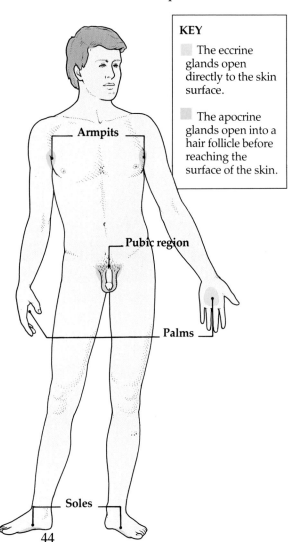

KEY
■ The eccrine glands open directly to the skin surface.

■ The apocrine glands open into a hair follicle before reaching the surface of the skin.

Armpits

Pubic region

Palms

Soles

The sweat glands
You have two types of sweat glands. The eccrine glands occur over most of your body, particularly on the palms and soles. The apocrine glands develop at puberty and are found in the armpits, in the pubic region, and around the anus. The production of sweat is one of the ways your body temperature is regulated. The bloodstream carries fluid into the sweat glands in your skin. Fluid then emerges from the glands as sweat. Heat is expended to evaporate this moisture, which helps cool the body. In extremes of heat or during vigorous exercise, you must lose more heat to maintain body temperature, so you sweat more.

MONITORING BOWEL AND URINARY HABITS

Each of us has a pattern of bowel or urinary activity that is "normal" for us. Most people usually have about one soft, formed bowel movement per day, but there is wide variation among healthy individuals, from one movement a week to three or four a day. The number of times that an individual usually empties his or her bladder varies similarly, depending on the amount of fluid consumed, the temperature, humidity, amount of clothing worn, and the amount of fluid lost in perspiration.

Staying alert to changes

In general, a change in your typical pattern of bowel or urinary activity may suggest a disorder. If your bowel movements become irregular, unusually infrequent, dry, or difficult to pass, you are probably suffering from constipation. Diarrhea describes the passage of excessive quantities of loose or liquid feces. Consult your doctor if constipation persists for more than 2 weeks or if diarrhea persists for more than 48 hours.

A change in the frequency of urination may be due to many causes – from diabetes or a bladder infection to benign obstruction of the prostate gland – and should be investigated by your doctor. Other symptoms that should prompt you to visit your doctor include an increase in the amount of urine, discomfort when passing urine, loss of small amounts of urine, or complete loss of bladder control.

Healthy feces vary widely in color and consistency. However, see your doctor if your feces appear pale gray, or if they become bulky, greasy, especially offensive-smelling, or tend to float. Blood in your stools is never normal. Consult your doctor if you experience bleeding during defecation or pass tar-like, black feces or feces containing bright red blood.

CAUSES OF ABNORMAL-LOOKING URINE

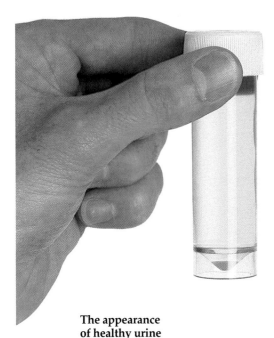

**The appearance
of healthy urine**
*Urine is usually clear and
straw-colored and has a
slight odor.*

APPEARANCE	POSSIBLE CAUSE
Pale yellow or colorless	Drinking a large quantity of liquid may temporarily make the diluted urine more pale in color, which is no cause for concern.
Darker, more concentrated yellow	Loss of fluid caused by sweating, vomiting, or diarrhea (if not replaced) may intensify the color of urine because of the reduction in the amount of water being excreted.
Yellow-orange to orange-red	Certain drugs, particularly laxatives containing senna, produce these color changes. If you are taking any form of medication, ask your doctor whether it may affect the color of your urine.
Brown	A liver or gallbladder disorder may cause broken-down blood products to enter the urine and darken it considerably. Your doctor should investigate any such color change.
Pink, red, or smoky brown	Certain drugs, food dyes, and produce such as black-berries or beets may redden the urine. However, a red color may also indicate blood in the urine. If you have any doubt as to the cause of this color change, show a sample of your urine to your doctor.
Excessively frothy	In kidney disorders that allow protein to leak through the kidneys into the urine, the urine may become excessively frothy. Consult your doctor if you notice such a change.

FECAL OCCULT BLOOD TESTING

Blood produced by gastrointestinal bleeding is not always visible in the feces. The presence of minute quantities of hidden (occult) blood in the feces can be detected by chemical tests. Your doctor may give you a special kit to collect a sample of feces. Do-it-yourself home fecal occult blood tests are also available over the counter. However, the interpretation of results is more accurate when done by medical personnel.

PROFESSIONAL URINE ANALYSIS

Urine may be tested in several ways to screen for kidney, urinary tract, and other diseases. Tests may be performed in the doctor's office or a laboratory. Substances in urine may be measured by simple biochemical tests or, more commonly today, by noting color changes in a chemically impregnated stick or strip dipped in urine. Examination of urine under a microscope is sometimes done to analyze or detect features such as those described below.

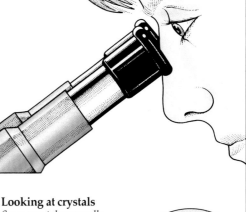

Looking at casts
Casts are proteinlike material that sometimes contain red blood cells, white blood cells, or other components. Casts in the urine con-firm the presence of kidney disease. The cast shown at right is as-sociated with heavy loss of protein.

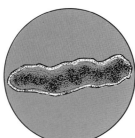

Looking at crystals
Some crystals normally appear in urine, but a high level of certain crystals may suggest a particular disorder. For example, uric acid crystals, shown at right, indicate an abnormally high level of uric acid in the urine.

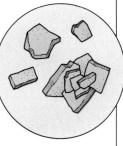

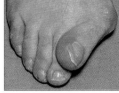

ARE YOUR FEET AND LEGS HEALTHY?

The lower parts of your legs and your feet carry the weight of your body and are strained if you are overweight or if you stand (but do not walk) for long periods. Varicose veins are a common problem in the legs, especially among women. These twisted, distended veins can be painful. Swollen ankles may be caused by being on your feet for a long time in warmer weather or by sitting with your feet tucked under your chair (such as during a long plane trip).

PROBLEMS THAT MAY AFFECT YOUR FEET

Most foot problems can be easily prevented by good foot care and hygiene and by making sure that your shoes fit well and provide good support.

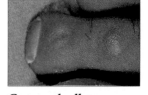

Corns and calluses
Calluses are hard areas of skin produced as a reaction to pressure or friction, usually from shoes that are too tight or fit poorly. A corn is a callus on a toe.

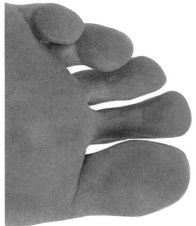

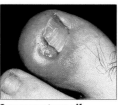

Athletes' foot
This fungal infection attacks the sole of your foot and the skin between your toes. It begins as a red, scaly, itchy rash. The skin may then crack and peel. The area may have an odor.

Plantar warts
Like all warts, plantar warts are caused by a virus infection of the skin. Because the wart grows on the underside of the foot, it is pushed inward and causes pain when standing and walking.

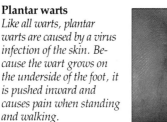

Ingrown toenail
This painful condition may occur if your nail is too wide for the nail bed, is under pressure from your shoes, or has been cut too short. An ingrown nail can easily become infected.

Bunion
This bump on the side of the big toe joint tends to make the toes point to the outside. It is largely a hereditary condition. If your parents have bunions, you are more likely to have them too.

DO YOU HAVE "FLAT FEET"?

Some people have feet that are naturally flat (that is, the foot lacks an arch so that the sole rests flat on the ground). In most cases, flat feet do not cause any problems. You can determine whether you have high- or low-arched feet by doing the following test using an ink pad.

Items needed

♦ Ink pad
♦ Piece of paper larger than your feet

Method

1 Place your foot on the ink pad or use a roller to cover the bottom of your foot with ink.

2 Carefully put your foot on the paper. Evenly distribute your weight between your feet.

3 Remove your foot from the paper, clean the ink from your foot, and repeat with your other foot. Check your results against the diagram.

High arch

Normal arch

Flat arch

However, they can also be a sign of a serious problem such as liver or kidney disease, or even heart failure. If unexplained swelling of your ankles persists, consult your doctor.

Many foot problems are the result of wearing badly fitting shoes or of poor foot hygiene. However, some problems may be due to a disorder affecting the circulation, such as arteriosclerosis. You also need to be alert to signs of skin cancer (shown on page 54).

Do you have varicose veins?
Varicose veins, shown below, are more common in women. They often occur after pregnancy. Early signs include swelling and aching and discoloration of the skin. If you have any of these signs, consult your doctor. He or she may advise you to wear support hose or an elastic bandage (see right).

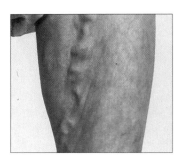

Monitoring the foot in diabetes
People with diabetes often lose their sensation of pain. As a result, they do not feel pressure points from badly fitting shoes that could be damaging their feet. In addition, their blood vessels tend to become blocked by atherosclerosis. Also, minor cuts and sores are slow to heal. Diabetes is the most common cause of amputation for gangrene (death of tissues). If you have diabetes, it is extremely important that you examine your feet regularly for problems, and get immediate medical attention if anything is wrong. If you think you might have trouble detecting any problems or if you have difficulty trimming your nails, get professional help with your foot care.

FOOT CARE FOR A PERSON WITH DIABETES
Be alert to sores, bruises, and cuts on your feet, which should be reported to your doctor immediately. Have your toenails cut regularly and any calluses pared and treated by your doctor or podiatrist. With good foot care you can prevent serious complications.

ASK YOUR DOCTOR YOUR GENERAL HEALTH

Q **I often wake up in the morning drenched in sweat. Is something wrong with me?**

A It may just be that your sheets or nightclothes are made of non-absorbent, synthetic materials. You'll be more comfortable in natural fibers such as cotton. For a woman between 35 and 50, sweating primarily at night is a common signal that the menopause is approaching. But night sweating is sometimes associated with infection. If your sweating is a recent change, consult your doctor.

Q **Over the last few weeks I've noticed that my ears feel "full." I am sure my hearing has been getting worse. I am only 27 – is it possible that I could be going deaf?**

A It is more likely that your ears have become blocked by earwax (cerumen). Your doctor will probably investigate this possibility first, before arranging for you to take some hearing tests. If wax is the problem, your doctor may use a syringe and warm water to flush your ears or he or she will instruct you on how to remove it yourself with drops made especially for this purpose.

Q **A month ago I tripped over a bucket and cut my leg below the knee. The cut still hasn't healed. Is there something wrong with my blood? I'm 50.**

A The skin that covers the shinbone is very thin, and cuts in this region heal slowly in middle-aged and older people. Consult your doctor so that the possibility of any circulatory problems can be excluded.

SYMPTOMS, SELF-MONITORING, AND TESTING

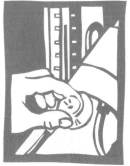

TODAY, PEOPLE ARE encouraged to take more responsibility for monitoring their health. You can be more actively involved in your health care – even when you feel fine – by being alert to warning symptoms and signs of disease, by performing self-examinations regularly, by having recommended medical tests, and, in some cases, by performing certain other tests at home.

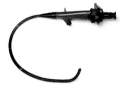

Sigmoidoscope
The sigmoidoscope is used to find benign polyps in the rectum and lower colon before they become malignant or to identify (at an early stage) polyps or tumors that have become malignant.

The purpose of many medical tests and self-examinations is to detect cancers at an early stage (when they can still be treated). It is also important to identify high blood pressure and raised blood cholesterol levels before complications develop. People already suffering from specific illnesses (such as asthma or diabetes) and those who are undergoing long-term drug treatment may need to have other health checkups. They, too, are encouraged to monitor their conditions as closely as possible.

PREVENTIVE HEALTH

It was once common to see your doctor only if you felt sick. We now know that an apparently healthy person can have a serious disease over a long period of time, during which there may be no overt signs or symptoms that anything is wrong. Seeing your doctor when you are not sick will help you establish a good doctor/patient relationship (which will ensure a better understanding of your

THE PAP SMEAR – A SUCCESS STORY

The cervical (Pap) smear has contributed remarkably to the prevention of cancer of the cervix. The test is quick and easy. If the results show unusual or cancerous change, treatment usually results in a complete cure. This test has reduced deaths from cervical cancer by up to 68 percent in the past 30 years.

Results of cervical screening
The graph shows the dramatic decrease in incidence of and mortality from cervical cancer in British Columbia, Canada, since the introduction of a cervical screening program. Mortality figures were not calculated before 1958.

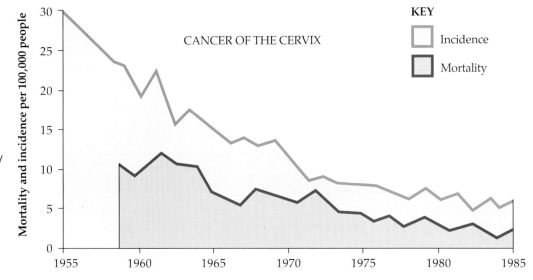

CANCER OF THE CERVIX

KEY
☐ Incidence
■ Mortality

SYMPTOMS AND SIGNS YOU SHOULD NOT IGNORE

You should be aware of the warning signs of potentially serious illness so that you will know when to consult your doctor. It would be impossible to include a comprehensive list of all diseases here so we have listed the symptoms and signs of the more commonly occurring, serious conditions. However, you should never ignore any other worrisome or persistent symptoms.

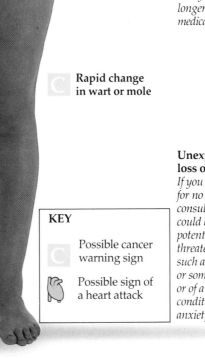

Loss of hearing
Sudden hearing loss, deafness, or ringing in the ears should always be checked by your doctor.

Chest pain that radiates to the neck and jaw or down one or both of your arms

Persistent cough or hoarseness

Disturbed or impaired vision
Any change in your eyesight, such as blurred vision, double vision, flashing lights or spots in front of the eyes, or loss of part or all of the field of vision, should be reported to your doctor immediately.

Lump in a breast or elsewhere

Unusual bleeding or discharge from genital tract or bleeding from urinary or digestive tract

Breathlessness when lying down that is relieved only by standing or sitting up

Persistent digestive complaints or difficulty swallowing

Fainting or dizzy spells
Isolated episodes of faintness or dizziness are not usually a cause for concern. However, if you faint repeatedly, seek medical advice.

Feelings of guilt and worthlessness
If your feelings of depression are so extreme that you feel that life is no longer worth living, seek medical help immediately.

Painful urination
This pain is usually the result of infection in the lower part of the urinary tract and should be treated immediately.

Change in bowel or bladder habits

Rapid change in wart or mole

Sore that does not heal

Clumsiness
Sudden onset of clumsiness in a previously well-coordinated person may be the result of a nervous or muscular system disorder and should be investigated.

Unexplained loss of weight
If you start to lose weight for no apparent reason, consult your doctor. It could be a sign of a potentially life-threatening condition, such as a serious infection or some types of cancer, or of a less threatening condition, such as anxiety.

KEY

Possible cancer warning sign

Possible sign of a heart attack

MONITOR YOUR SYMPTOMS
ABDOMINAL PAIN

Pain in the abdomen may be experienced as a generalized feeling of discomfort in the entire region below your rib cage or as a specific pain in one spot. A minor digestive upset may cause the sudden onset of abdominal pain. However, persistent, severe abdominal pain is always reason to see your doctor promptly. Recurrent abdominal pain has different causes and is not addressed here.

WARNING

Seek immediate medical attention if your abdominal pain:

◆ Persists for more than 4 hours
◆ Is accompanied but unrelieved (even temporarily) by vomiting
◆ Is accompanied by faintness, drowsiness, or confusion

KEY ♂ Men ♀ Women

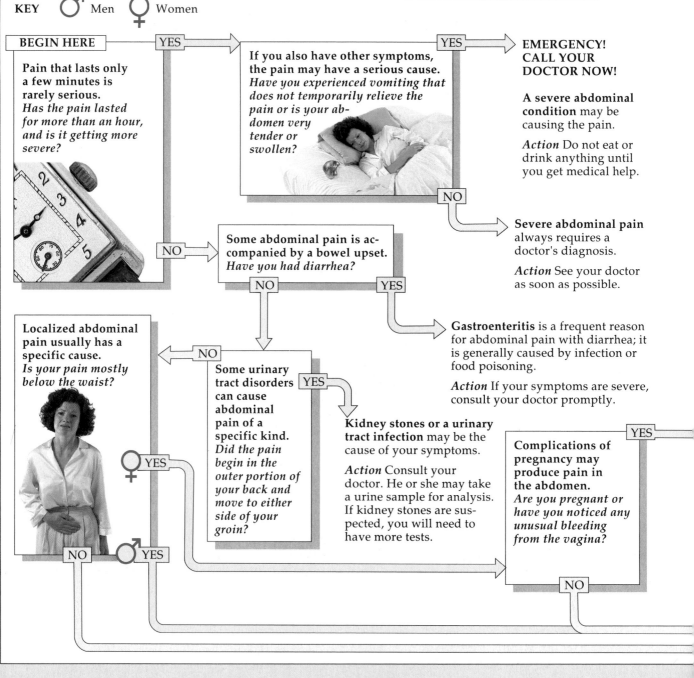

BEGIN HERE — YES →

Pain that lasts only a few minutes is rarely serious.
Has the pain lasted for more than an hour, and is it getting more severe?

If you also have other symptoms, the pain may have a serious cause.
Have you experienced vomiting that does not temporarily relieve the pain or is your abdomen very tender or swollen?

— YES →

EMERGENCY! CALL YOUR DOCTOR NOW!

A severe abdominal condition may be causing the pain.

Action Do not eat or drink anything until you get medical help.

NO →

Severe abdominal pain always requires a doctor's diagnosis.

Action See your doctor as soon as possible.

NO →

Some abdominal pain is accompanied by a bowel upset.
Have you had diarrhea?

NO / YES

Gastroenteritis is a frequent reason for abdominal pain with diarrhea; it is generally caused by infection or food poisoning.

Action If your symptoms are severe, consult your doctor promptly.

Localized abdominal pain usually has a specific cause.
Is your pain mostly below the waist?

NO ←

Some urinary tract disorders can cause abdominal pain of a specific kind.
Did the pain begin in the outer portion of your back and move to either side of your groin?

YES →

Kidney stones or a urinary tract infection may be the cause of your symptoms.

Action Consult your doctor. He or she may take a urine sample for analysis. If kidney stones are suspected, you will need to have more tests.

♀ YES

♂ YES

NO

Complications of pregnancy may produce pain in the abdomen.
Are you pregnant or have you noticed any unusual bleeding from the vagina?

YES

NO

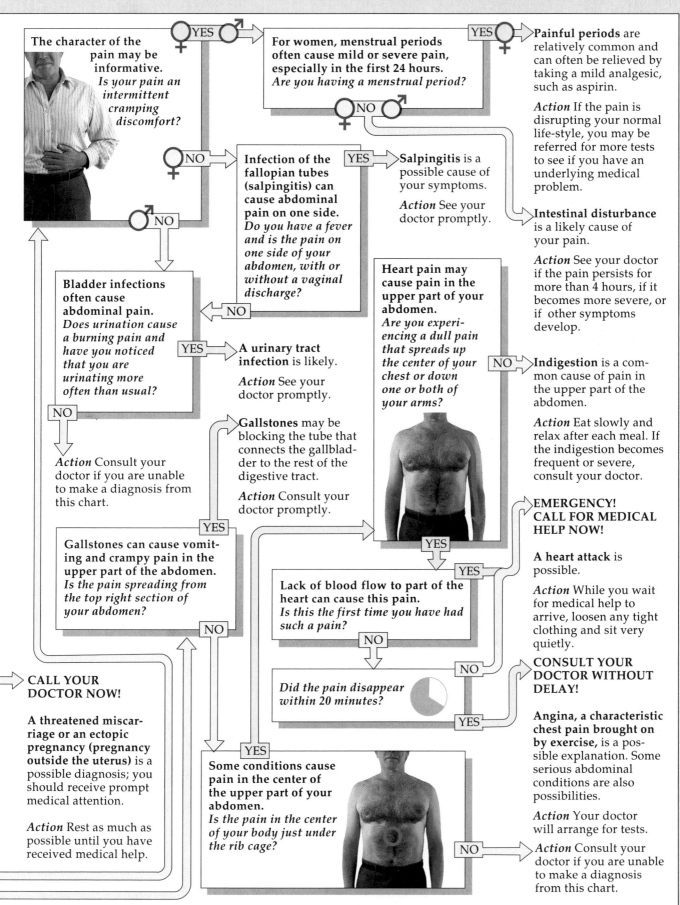

The character of the pain may be informative. *Is your pain an intermittent cramping discomfort?*

YES ♀ ♂

For women, menstrual periods often cause mild or severe pain, especially in the first 24 hours. *Are you having a menstrual period?*

YES ♀

Painful periods are relatively common and can often be relieved by taking a mild analgesic, such as aspirin.

Action If the pain is disrupting your normal life-style, you may be referred for more tests to see if you have an underlying medical problem.

NO ♂ ♀

NO ♀

Infection of the fallopian tubes (salpingitis) can cause abdominal pain on one side. *Do you have a fever and is the pain on one side of your abdomen, with or without a vaginal discharge?*

YES

Salpingitis is a possible cause of your symptoms.

Action See your doctor promptly.

Intestinal disturbance is a likely cause of your pain.

Action See your doctor if the pain persists for more than 4 hours, if it becomes more severe, or if other symptoms develop.

NO ♂

NO

Bladder infections often cause abdominal pain. *Does urination cause a burning pain and have you noticed that you are urinating more often than usual?*

YES

A urinary tract infection is likely.

Action See your doctor promptly.

Heart pain may cause pain in the upper part of your abdomen. *Are you experiencing a dull pain that spreads up the center of your chest or down one or both of your arms?*

NO

Indigestion is a common cause of pain in the upper part of the abdomen.

Action Eat slowly and relax after each meal. If the indigestion becomes frequent or severe, consult your doctor.

NO

Action Consult your doctor if you are unable to make a diagnosis from this chart.

Gallstones may be blocking the tube that connects the gallbladder to the rest of the digestive tract.

Action Consult your doctor promptly.

YES

EMERGENCY! CALL FOR MEDICAL HELP NOW!

A heart attack is possible.

Action While you wait for medical help to arrive, loosen any tight clothing and sit very quietly.

YES

Gallstones can cause vomiting and crampy pain in the upper part of the abdomen. *Is the pain spreading from the top right section of your abdomen?*

YES

Lack of blood flow to part of the heart can cause this pain. *Is this the first time you have had such a pain?*

YES

NO

CONSULT YOUR DOCTOR WITHOUT DELAY!

NO

NO

Did the pain disappear within 20 minutes?

YES

CALL YOUR DOCTOR NOW!

A threatened miscarriage or an ectopic pregnancy (pregnancy outside the uterus) is a possible diagnosis; you should receive prompt medical attention.

Action Rest as much as possible until you have received medical help.

Angina, a characteristic chest pain brought on by exercise, is a possible explanation. Some serious abdominal conditions are also possibilities.

Action Your doctor will arrange for tests.

YES

Some conditions cause pain in the center of the upper part of your abdomen. *Is the pain in the center of your body just under the rib cage?*

NO

Action Consult your doctor if you are unable to make a diagnosis from this chart.

state of health). You and your doctor can discuss ways you can improve your health. Your doctor also may suggest tests to look for "silent" conditions, some of which may run in your family.

To be of value, screening tests need to fulfill certain conditions. They must be reasonably accurate, with a minimum of false-positive results (cases incorrectly diagnosed) and false-negative results (missed diagnoses). They also must be simple to administer, acceptable to the patient, and inexpensive enough that they can be done for many people. Effective treatment must be available for the diseases the tests are designed to detect. Finally, evidence must indicate that early treatment improves the chance of cure.

Choice and timing of tests

The types of tests and the frequency with which you have them done depend on several factors. Your age and sex are important; your medical history must be taken into account; and certain family histories, occupations, and habits that put you in a special risk category may justify individualized testing.

The recommended tests are shown in the chart on page 17. If you think you might need other tests because of special factors, talk to your doctor.

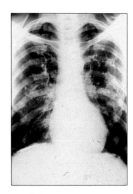

Looking for asbestosis
People who have worked with asbestos are at risk of asbestosis (solidification and scarring of lung tissue) and need to have regular evaluation with chest X-rays.

CANCER SELF-EXAMINATIONS

Because you are most familiar with your body, you are in the best position to detect any abnormal changes that might be early warning signs of cancer. In addition to having the recommended cancer screening tests, you should also make a point of examining your skin and breasts or testicles regularly.

TESTICLE SELF-EXAMINATION

Men between the ages of 20 and 40 should perform a self-examination of their testicles about once a month to look for lumps or swellings that may indicate cancer. Testicular cancer is the most common cancer in young men. If detected early, it is one of the most easily curable of all cancers, so self-examination (in addition to your doctor's periodic examinations) is worthwhile. The best time to perform the examination is during or after a bath or shower when the scrotal skin is relaxed.

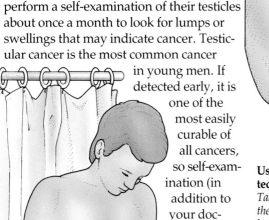

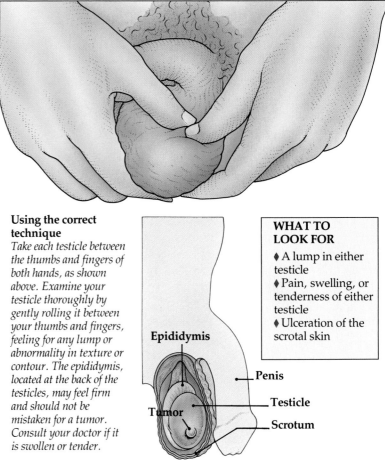

Using the correct technique
Take each testicle between the thumbs and fingers of both hands, as shown above. Examine your testicle thoroughly by gently rolling it between your thumbs and fingers, feeling for any lump or abnormality in texture or contour. The epididymis, located at the back of the testicles, may feel firm and should not be mistaken for a tumor. Consult your doctor if it is swollen or tender.

Epididymis

Tumor

Penis

Testicle

Scrotum

WHAT TO LOOK FOR
♦ A lump in either testicle
♦ Pain, swelling, or tenderness of either testicle
♦ Ulceration of the scrotal skin

BREAST SELF-EXAMINATION

Every woman over age 20 should perform a monthly breast self-examination so that she is acquainted with the normal characteristics of her breasts and will have a better chance of noticing any changes. The best time to examine yourself is at the end of your period when your breasts are usually not tender and are likely to be the least lumpy. After menopause, you can examine your breasts any time of the month, provided that you do it at the same time each month. Report any unusual change to your doctor immediately.

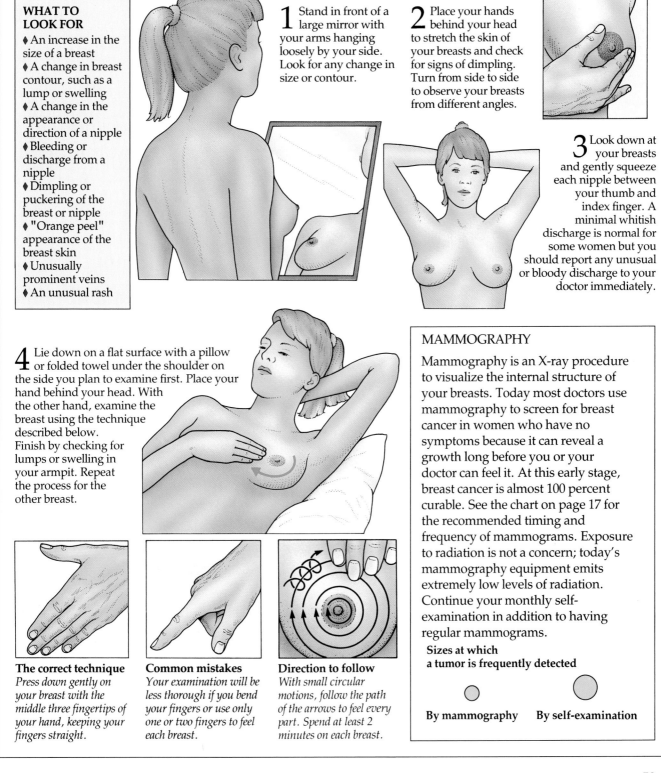

WHAT TO LOOK FOR

♦ An increase in the size of a breast
♦ A change in breast contour, such as a lump or swelling
♦ A change in the appearance or direction of a nipple
♦ Bleeding or discharge from a nipple
♦ Dimpling or puckering of the breast or nipple
♦ "Orange peel" appearance of the breast skin
♦ Unusually prominent veins
♦ An unusual rash

1 Stand in front of a large mirror with your arms hanging loosely by your side. Look for any change in size or contour.

2 Place your hands behind your head to stretch the skin of your breasts and check for signs of dimpling. Turn from side to side to observe your breasts from different angles.

3 Look down at your breasts and gently squeeze each nipple between your thumb and index finger. A minimal whitish discharge is normal for some women but you should report any unusual or bloody discharge to your doctor immediately.

4 Lie down on a flat surface with a pillow or folded towel under the shoulder on the side you plan to examine first. Place your hand behind your head. With the other hand, examine the breast using the technique described below. Finish by checking for lumps or swelling in your armpit. Repeat the process for the other breast.

The correct technique
Press down gently on your breast with the middle three fingertips of your hand, keeping your fingers straight.

Common mistakes
Your examination will be less thorough if you bend your fingers or use only one or two fingers to feel each breast.

Direction to follow
With small circular motions, follow the path of the arrows to feel every part. Spend at least 2 minutes on each breast.

MAMMOGRAPHY

Mammography is an X-ray procedure to visualize the internal structure of your breasts. Today most doctors use mammography to screen for breast cancer in women who have no symptoms because it can reveal a growth long before you or your doctor can feel it. At this early stage, breast cancer is almost 100 percent curable. See the chart on page 17 for the recommended timing and frequency of mammograms. Exposure to radiation is not a concern; today's mammography equipment emits extremely low levels of radiation. Continue your monthly self-examination in addition to having regular mammograms.

Sizes at which a tumor is frequently detected

By mammography   By self-examination

53

SKIN SELF-EXAMINATION

The American Cancer Society recommends that everyone perform a regular self-examination of the skin to detect early signs of skin cancer. Cancer of the skin is the most common form of the disease, and it is also the easiest to detect. Most skin cancers are completely curable if discovered at an early stage. If you have a fair complexion and are over 30, self-examination is particularly important – especially if you have been exposed to the sun without protection for prolonged periods.

HOW TO EXAMINE YOUR SKIN

Perform your examination in a well-lighted room in front of a full-length mirror. First inspect your skin in general, looking for any changes and counting your moles. Make a "mole map" as shown in the illustration at right. Each time you do your examination, refer to the map to see whether any new moles have appeared.

Now do a detailed examination, starting at your head and working down. Use a hand mirror to look at inaccessible areas and a magnifying glass to check suspicious-looking moles. All sun-exposed areas need to be examined particularly carefully.

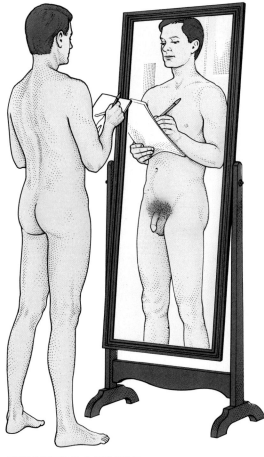

Making a "mole map"
Draw outlines of the front and back of your body (or photocopy the outlines provided on page 138) and draw your most prominent moles on the "map" or ask someone to do it for you.

CHECKLIST OF AREAS TO EXAMINE
◆ Face and neck. If you are a man, check under your facial hair.
◆ Scalp. Part your hair (or use a blow dryer) to permit you to take a close look.
◆ Arms (including the backs of your upper arms) and shoulders.
◆ Back and buttocks.
◆ Back of legs.
◆ Front of legs and all parts of the feet, including the soles.
◆ Under your fingernails and toenails. Look for dark spots, which could indicate malignant melanoma.

WHAT TO LOOK FOR

◆ Change in skin color or texture
◆ A sore that does not heal in 3 weeks
◆ Any mole or blemish that changes in appearance, grows, itches, or bleeds

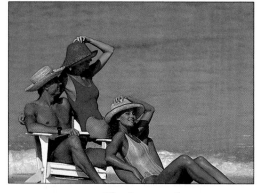

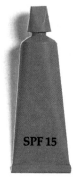

The dangers of sun exposure
In the US, almost all of the more than 500,000 cases of nonmelanoma skin cancers that occur each year are thought to be related to sun exposure. Exposure to the sun's ultraviolet rays is also a major factor in the development of malignant melanoma, a less common but more serious condition. If you spend a great deal of time in the sun, use a sunscreen with a sun protection factor (SPF) of 15 or higher.

SPF 15

HOW TO RECOGNIZE A MALIGNANT MELANOMA

Melanoma tends to spread to other parts of the body, including the vital organs, which makes it a lethal form of cancer. A melanoma has characteristics that distinguish it from a normal mole. Use the ABCD checklist below to help you remember the danger signs.

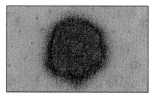

Normal mole
(Magnification × 2.5)
Almost symmetrical; round or oval. Definite border and flat or evenly raised surface. Usually tan to dark brown and evenly pigmented.

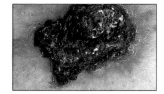

Malignant melanoma
(Magnification × 1.5)
Asymmetrical.
Border – irregular or unclear.
Color – not uniform; may include tan, brown, blue, black, or red.
Diameter – greater than ¼ inch.

BLOOD PRESSURE CHECKUPS

Uncontrolled high blood pressure (hypertension) damages your heart and arteries and increases your risk of a number of serious diseases. Strokes, heart attacks, kidney failure, and eye damage can ultimately result from untreated hypertension. About 23 million Americans have high blood pressure; only about half of these people know they have it. Hypertension causes no symptoms, so everyone should have his or her blood pressure checked regularly. You should have a checkup at age 20. If it is normal, you need to be checked at 3- to 5-year intervals. However, it is easy to have your blood pressure checked every time you visit your doctor. If your blood pressure is high, your doctor will advise you about diet, exercise, and control of factors such as smoking, drinking, and the level of stress in your life. Your doctor may prescribe medication.

MEASURING BLOOD PRESSURE

Blood pressure is the pressure the blood exerts on the walls of the blood vessels. The pressure wave is measured at its maximum when the heart has just contracted (systolic pressure) and at its minimum between heart beats (diastolic pressure). These measurements are expressed in millimeters of mercury (mm Hg), as systolic over diastolic (the systolic reading is given first). A reading higher than 150 systolic or 90 diastolic is generally considered high.

MONITORING YOUR BLOOD PRESSURE

If your blood pressure cannot be controlled satisfactorily, or if it varies with each checkup despite treatment, your doctor may ask you to monitor it yourself. Taking your own blood pressure has several advantages. You can take readings at different times of the day and, because you are in familiar surroundings, there may be less chance that the pressure will be artificially elevated by anxiety. You may be asked to take your blood pressure at regular intervals over several months. Rest for 5 minutes before taking the measurement. Report your home measurements to your doctor. The instrument used to measure blood pressure is called a sphygmomanometer. Various models are available for home use. Some devices have an electronic sensor and incorporate a microphone instead of a stethoscope in the cuff; they are slightly less accurate.

1 Place the cuff around your arm just above the elbow. Place the head of the stethoscope over your artery on the inner side of your arm just below the elbow. You can buckle the cuff of some models snugly around your arm (shown right).

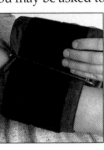

2 Inflate the cuff to just above your systolic pressure. This will be about 20 millimeters higher than where you expect the systolic pressure reading to be (based on your earlier checkups).

3 Now deflate the cuff slowly while you listen through the stethoscope.

4 When you hear the first sound, record the pressure indicated on the gauge. This reading is the systolic pressure.

5 Continue deflating the cuff. When all sound ceases, take another reading. This figure is the diastolic pressure.

Pressure gauge

Cuff

Head of the stethoscope

Bulb for inflating cuff

CHOLESTEROL CHECKUPS

Cholesterol is the best known of the lipids, a group of essential fatty substances found in all body cells and in the blood. Many people in developed countries have more cholesterol in their blood than is healthy. Research has shown convincingly that, when people who have high blood cholesterol levels modify their diets and successfully lower their levels, they reduce their risk of having heart attacks or strokes.

Who should be checked?

All adults should have their cholesterol levels checked regularly. Your cholesterol level should be checked once in childhood and then every 5 years after age 20. The results of the last checkup will determine the frequency of future testing. The cholesterol test requires only a small blood sample.

What happens after the test?

If at any age your cholesterol level is found to be more than 200 milligrams per deciliter (mg/dL), the first step is to have another test to confirm the accuracy. If your cholesterol level is 200 to 239 mg/dL and you have no other risk factors for heart disease (such as smoking, diabetes, high blood pressure, history of disease in the family, or obesity), you will probably be given general advice on how to modify your diet and increase your level of exercise. If your cholesterol level is 200 to 239 mg/dL and you have two or more risk factors, or your cholesterol level is more than 240 mg/dL, your doctor will measure the levels of other lipids in your blood, such as high-density lipoprotein, low-density lipoprotein, and triglycerides. The results of these tests help determine treatment. A low-fat, low-cholesterol, high-fiber diet is almost always the first step. If the dietary changes fail to lower your cholesterol level or if your cholesterol level is very high, medication may be needed as well.

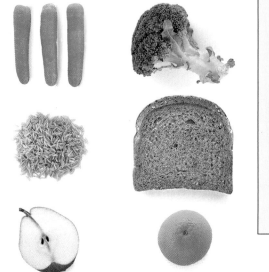

Diet and your cholesterol level
Reducing the amount of fat, particularly saturated fat, in your diet is an important means of reducing your cholesterol level. Current recommendations are that less than 30 percent of your calorie intake be derived from fat (and no more than 10 percent from saturated fat). Most of your calories should come from fruits, vegetables, and grains.

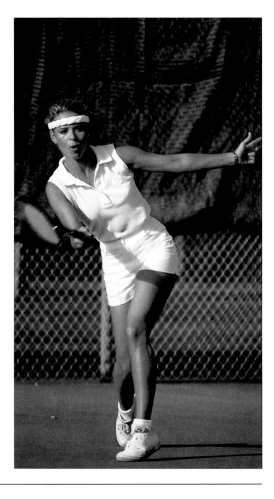

Exercise and your cholesterol level
Exercising helps you lose weight and thus contributes to a reduction in your cholesterol level. Regular aerobic exercise may also increase your high-density lipoproteins, which offer protection against heart disease.

WHAT IS THE NORMAL BLOOD CHOLESTEROL LEVEL?

Normal blood cholesterol levels vary among healthy people as do other differences such as weight and blood pressure. However, the higher the cholesterol level, the greater the risk of coronary heart disease and stroke.

CASE HISTORY
AN INFECTED FOOT

FRAN HAD BEEN ON **her feet more than usual because the museum where she works had opened a new wing. One night after an opening, she noticed calluses on her left foot, so she trimmed them away with manicure scissors. Fran tried to be careful but she cut too deeply and her foot bled. When the area became inflamed and tender a few days later, she called her doctor.**

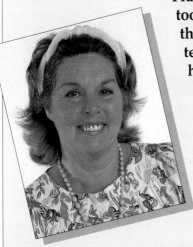

PERSONAL DETAILS
Name Fran Tressler
Age 57
Occupation Fund-raiser for an art museum
Family Fran's mother and one of her sisters have diabetes.

MEDICAL BACKGROUND
Fran was diagnosed as having non-insulin-dependent diabetes when she was 35 years old. She has successfully kept her blood sugar level down by regulating her diet. She knows she should exercise more often to keep her weight down and to help maintain good circulation, but she cannot seem to find the time. Lately, she has noticed that her feet occasionally feel numb.

THE DIAGNOSIS
The doctor notices pus coming from the cut on her foot so he takes a sample to send to the laboratory for a bacterial culture. The results show that Fran has a STAPHYLOCOCCAL IN-FECTION. The infection would be less serious in a person with a normal blood sugar level. For Fran, however, the problem is more threatening because she is likely to get infections more easily and to have a harder time fighting the infections. Also, her impaired circulation will slow the healing process.

THE TREATMENT
Fran's doctor is concerned and prescribes an antibiotic and a mild antiseptic solution for the infection. He asks her to stay off her feet and to keep her infected foot elevated until the infection is gone and the cut has healed. The doctor warns Fran that long-term, uncontrolled diabetes is the most common reason for amputation of the feet and legs. Because of her diabetes and her age, the small arteries in her legs are narrowing and are

Professional foot care
Fran's doctor advises her not to cut or trim her toenails or calluses by herself. She now regularly visits her doctor's office for care of her feet.

not able to carry the necessary amounts of blood, oxygen, and infection-fighting white cells to her feet. Prevention of injury and infection is more important than ever. Her doctor instructs her to bathe her foot in warm water and the antiseptic solution twice a day, to examine her foot closely for any signs that the infection is spreading, and to notify him immediately if problems develop. He also tells her to throw out the poorly fitting shoes that seem to have caused the calluses. Most importantly, he tells her to set up regular appointments to have her toenails and calluses trimmed in his office.

THE OUTCOME
Fran remains off her feet for almost 6 weeks until her foot has healed. She is extremely careful to shop for shoes that fit and to break them in gradually before wearing them all day. She does not try to cut or trim her toenails or calluses by herself.

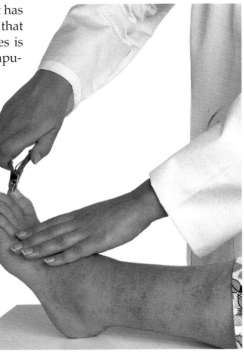

MONITORING LONG-TERM DRUG TREATMENT

If you are undergoing long-term drug treatment for a medical problem, you should always take the correct amount of medication at the correct times (as recommended by your doctor). You also need to watch for potential side effects that may or may not have serious consequences. Some of the most common long-term medications are for treatment of high blood pressure and early heart disease. Two examples of these medications are described here.

THIAZIDE DIURETICS FOR HIGH BLOOD PRESSURE

Side effects you may encounter that do not usually require emergency medical attention
- Unusual tiredness when first starting to take the medication
- An increase in frequency of urination and amount of urine
- Decreased sexual ability
- Increased skin sensitivity to sunlight
- Loss of appetite, upset stomach, or diarrhea

Side effects that you should report to your doctor immediately
- Irregular heartbeat
- Loss of muscle strength
- Rash, such as hives
- Sore throat and fever
- Severe stomach pain, nausea, and vomiting
- Unusual bleeding or bruising
- Yellow eyes or skin
- Dizziness or light-headedness when standing

BETA BLOCKERS FOR EARLY HEART DISEASE

Side effects you may encounter that do not usually require emergency medical attention
- Decreased sexual ability
- Dizziness or light-headedness
- Slight drowsiness
- Insomnia
- Unusual tiredness or weakness
- Nightmares and vivid dreams

Side effects that you should report to your doctor immediately
- Breathing difficulty, irregular heartbeat, or slow pulse
- Cold hands and feet
- Confusion, hallucinations, or depression
- Swelling of ankles, feet, or lower legs
- Fever and sore throat
- Rash or red, scaling, or crusted skin
- Unusual bleeding and bruising

WARNING
Do not suddenly stop taking a beta blocker. You could experience a severe recurrence of your previous symptoms, your blood pressure could rise significantly, or you could have a heart attack. If your doctor determines that you should stop taking this medication, he or she will decrease your dosage gradually.

MONITORING DIABETES

If you have diabetes, your health depends on how well you control the disease. People who have diabetes are prone to coronary heart disease, stroke, kidney disease, eye problems (including cataracts and retinal damage), and neuropathies (damage to the nerves). Some evidence suggests that these risks are reduced if you keep your blood sugar level close to normal.

Maintenance of a nearly normal blood sugar level requires careful attention to the timing and size of your meals and the amount you exercise. You should learn how to measure your blood glucose level. With your doctor you can "fine-tune" your dosage of insulin or oral medications and take into account variations in your life-style, such as physical exertion and travel.

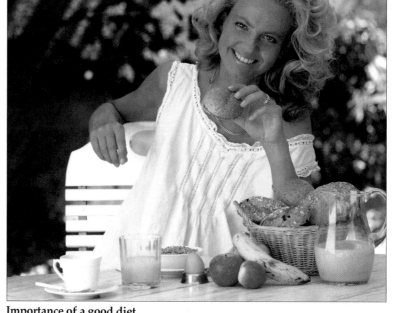

Importance of a good diet
If you have diabetes, it is important not to eat many sugar-containing foods (unless you are having a hypoglycemic attack). Instead you should get the carbohydrates you need from high-fiber grains, fruits, and vegetables. Some good substitutes for sugar-rich foods are shown above.

MEASURING BLOOD GLUCOSE LEVEL

You can measure your blood glucose level indirectly by testing your urine or directly by testing your blood. Urine tests are easy to perform but they tell you only when your blood glucose level is too high, not when it is too low. Blood tests are more complicated to perform but tell you more precisely what your blood sugar level is.

FREQUENCY OF TESTING

How often you test depends on your treatment, how well your diabetes is controlled, and how much time you are prepared to give. The frequency of your tests should be based on your doctor's advice. You may be asked to test more often if your blood sugar level fluctuates widely.

TESTING YOUR BLOOD

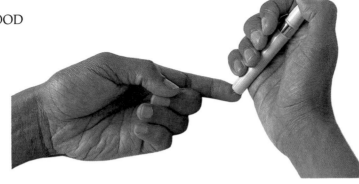

1 Obtain a drop of blood by pricking your finger or by using a special device (as shown) that pricks it automatically. The sides of your fingertips, your thumb, and your fourth finger are the least sensitive to pain.

2 Make sure the drop of blood you draw is large enough to cover the chemically treated area of the testing strip.

3 Hold the testing strip horizontally and thoroughly apply the blood sample.

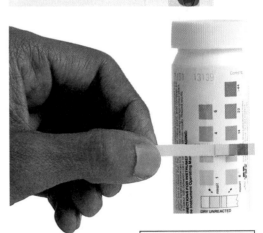

4 To determine your blood glucose level, compare the color of the strip with the color scale provided on the container (as shown). Or you can use an automatic device that will read the color.

URINE TESTING

Urine is tested by adding a special tablet to a sample of urine in a test tube and noting the color change, or by dipping a chemically treated strip into a urine sample and watching for a color change.

How to test your urine
Place a sample of urine in a test tube according to the manufacturer's directions. Add the special tablet and observe the color change (shown right).

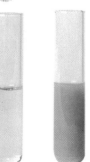

Time / Date	Urine/Glucose			Remarks:
	8am	2:30 pm	6pm	10 pm	
Mon	6/25/90 neg			
Tue	6/26/90 neg			
Wed	6/27/90	++		After meal
Thur	6/28/90 neg			
Fri	6/29/90		neg	
Sat				
Sun	7/1/90			Heavy meal/night

Recording the results
Record your results on a chart, such as the one shown here. After a few weeks, you will recognize a pattern in the times when your blood sugar levels are high. Take the charts with you when you see your doctor for a checkup. Your doctor may use this information to adjust your medication or modify your diet.

TESTING FOR KETONES

If your blood glucose level is very high or very low, you may want to test for substances called ketones in your urine. The method is similar to that used for testing glucose in urine. If ketones are present and your blood glucose level is high, contact your doctor immediately so that he or she can alter your treatment and bring down your blood glucose level.

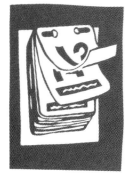

MENSTRUATION AND MENOPAUSE

MENSTRUATION IS THE NORMAL periodic loss of blood and uterine lining, by way of the vagina, in a woman who is not pregnant. The flow usually lasts 4 to 5 days and recurs about every 28 days. Menstruation starts with puberty and continues for about 30 years in most women. The first menstrual period is called the menarche and the ending of menstruation is called the menopause.

In developed countries, the menarche usually occurs at 12 or 13 years of age. However, some girls start having periods as early as 9 or as late as 16. The age of onset of menstruation depends on many factors, both genetic and environmental. It is closely associated with body weight and usually occurs when the girl or young woman has reached a weight of at least 84 to 88 pounds. Improved nutrition, better standards of general health, and earlier attainment of the adolescent growth spurt are the primary factors that have led to a gradual lowering of the age of onset of menstruation in many socio-economically advantaged countries.

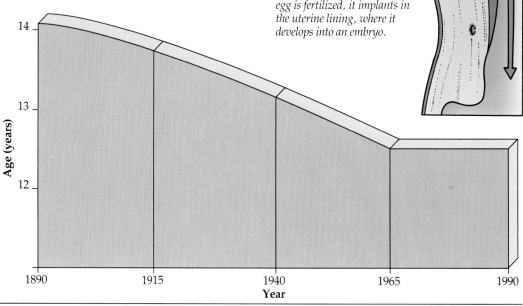

Egg

Ovary

Uterine lining

Uterus

Ovulation
A woman is born with about 1 million immature egg cells (ova) in each of her ovaries. Only one egg is released each month during ovulation; this occurs at about mid-cycle. If the egg is not fertilized by a male sperm cell, it passes out of the uterus along with the uterine lining. If the egg is fertilized, it implants in the uterine lining, where it develops into an embryo.

Onset of menstruation
In developed countries, the average age of onset of menstruation dropped by about 3 months each decade since the 1890s, until leveling off around 1965. Girls menstruate sooner now because of better nutrition and standards of health. The age of onset of menstruation is closely associated with body weight. The graph shows the decline in the mean age of the onset of menstruation for girls in the US. The 1890 figure is based on a report of patients at a clinic.

Age (years)

14

13

12

1890   1915   1940   1965   1990
Year

Hormone changes during the menstrual cycle
When a pituitary hormone stimulates the ripening of an egg in the ovary, estrogen levels rise, and the uterus lining (endometrium) thickens. The egg travels through the fallopian tubes into the uterus. Progesterone levels rise. If the egg is not fertilized, progesterone levels fall and the egg and the lining are shed.

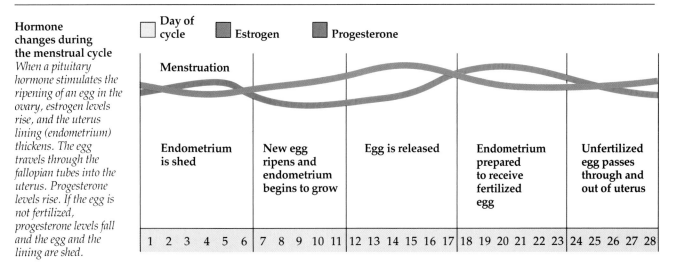

☐ Day of cycle   ▨ Estrogen   ▨ Progesterone

Menstruation

Endometrium is shed	New egg ripens and endometrium begins to grow	Egg is released	Endometrium prepared to receive fertilized egg	Unfertilized egg passes through and out of uterus
1 2 3 4 5 6	7 8 9 10 11	12 13 14 15 16 17	18 19 20 21 22 23	24 25 26 27 28

Most women reach the menopause around the age of 50, but it may occur as early as 40 or as late as 55. Just as the age of onset of menstruation is getting lower, so the age of the menopause is rising, for reasons that are not understood.

MONITORING MENSTRUATION

Menstruation is a natural, healthy aspect of a woman's life cycle, defining her fertile years. The menstrual period is the end result of a series of hormonal interactions in your body. You will experience some normal variations and everyday problems in your menstrual cycle. More serious complications can arise as a result of such factors as pregnancy in a very young girl or the long-term use of oral contraceptives.

The start of menstruation
At the onset of menstruation, periods are irregular in length and are usually relatively painless. The amount of blood loss varies. After regular ovulation begins, you can expect that your menstrual periods will become more regular.

In the early, irregular cycles around the time of puberty, ovulation may not occur. However, a young girl cannot assume that she will not become pregnant. Anemia and many other serious complications of pregnancy are more likely to develop in very young girls.

PREMENSTRUAL SYNDROME

More than 90 percent of women are aware of changes – minor to very severe – that sometimes occur in the few days before menstruation. Emotional symptoms include depression, anxiety, tension, irritability, and fatigue. Physical changes include fullness and tenderness of the breasts, lower abdominal discomfort or pain, fluid retention, muscular tension, constipation, clumsiness, and headache. If your premenstrual problems are severe, ask your doctor for advice.

Menstrual stages
A girl may start menstruating any time between 9 and 16, and continue for approximately 30 years. The climacteric is the term for the time span during which a woman moves from her reproductive to her nonreproductive stage. The 10- to 15-year period during which hormonal changes occur and menstrual flow gradually ceases is known as the premenopausal stage. The time of the last period is the menopause. It usually occurs between 48 and 55.

Menarche (onset of menstruation)   Premenopausal stage   Menopause (last menstrual period)

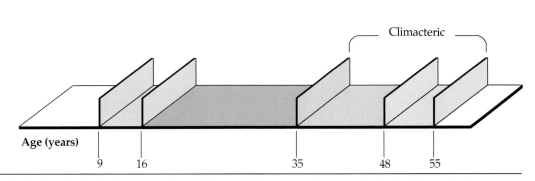

Climacteric

Age (years)

9   16   35   48   55

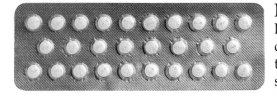

The pill
The hormones in oral contraceptives effectively "take over" the natural hormonal control of menstruation. Women who take oral contraceptives typically have lighter, shorter, and very regular periods.

The normal menstrual flow

The length of the period varies among healthy women from 2 to 7 days. The volume of blood and uterine lining (endometrium) lost during each period also varies considerably. The average loss of blood is about 2 fluid ounces but the amount may vary from 1 ounce to 6 ounces. Menstrual blood does not clot because of the absence of fibrinogen, an ingredient essential for blood clotting. However, the passage of lumps of compacted blood and tissue is common.

Menstrual problems

Dysmenorrhea – painful menstruation caused by powerful muscular contractions of the uterus (cramps) – was once a serious disorder for many women. It can now be effectively treated in up to 90 percent of cases with combined estrogen-progesterone oral contraceptives. An alternate treatment is with drugs that block the effects of prostaglandins, the substances that cause the painful contractions.

Irregular cycles should be evaluated by your doctor. The condition may be linked with weight loss or gain, stress, or illness. Oral contraceptives can be used to control irregular cycles.

Amenorrhea is the absence of menstrual periods. If your periods stop and you are not pregnant, possible causes include abrupt weight change, severe stress, excessive exercise (more than 20 to 40 miles of running per week), or problems with your pituitary or thyroid gland.

MENSTRUAL DISORDERS

Consult your doctor if you experience any of the following symptoms:

♦ Excessively painful periods
♦ Excessive amount and duration of menstrual blood loss
♦ Unusually light menstrual blood loss
♦ Absence of periods (if you are not pregnant)
♦ Bleeding from the uterus at irregular intervals
♦ Periods at intervals of less than 18 days
♦ Periods at intervals of more than 45 days
♦ Bleeding between normal periods

Administering estrogen
Estrogen is most commonly prescribed in pill form but vaginal creams or ointments containing estrogen may also be used to combat dryness and thinning of the skin of the vagina. Estrogen may also be administered through the skin by applying an adhesive patch, as shown.

ESTROGEN REPLACEMENT THERAPY

If you are approaching the menopause, discuss the risks and benefits of estrogen replacement therapy with your doctor. Administered over a period of years, estrogen can relieve unpleasant symptoms related to reduced estrogen levels. For women at high risk of osteoporosis, long-term therapy substantially reduces the chances of bone fracture. In addition, some studies show that estrogen lowers the risk of cardiovascular disease, and some evidence suggests that women taking estrogen suffer from depression less often.

Estrogen replacement therapy is not appropriate for everyone. Taking estrogen alone causes a slight increase in the risk of cancer of the uterus. But when progestin, a synthetic form of progesterone, is given in addition to estrogen, this risk is reduced. However, combination therapy causes continuation of periodic spotting. Estrogen replacement therapy is not recommended for women who have a history of breast or uterine cancer. It is also not suitable for women with a history of stroke, pulmonary embolism, deep-vein thrombosis, or liver disease. Taking estrogen may lead to minor side effects such as breast discomfort, water retention, and nausea.

MENOPAUSE

You probably cannot predict when your menopause will occur. Studies have not demonstrated any reliable relationship between the age of the onset of menstruation and the age of menopause. Some research suggests that factors such as use of oral contraceptives, childbearing experience, and obesity may influence age of menopause, but these associations are not fully understood.

The first sign of the approach of the menopause is a change in the pattern of your menstrual cycle. At first the cycle usually gets shorter – often by as much as a week – and then it tends to lengthen, with smaller, shorter, bleeding periods. A woman may have no periods for several months and then resume having irregular periods for a while. After 2 or 3 years or more of such irregularity, menstruation stops altogether.

During many of these later cycles, a woman does not ovulate. It is believed that, in women 40 to 45, a quarter of the cycles do not involve the release of an egg. After 45, the proportion of cycles without ovulation increases, so the chances of pregnancy are reduced.

Altered hormone production

As a woman approaches the age of menopause, her body produces less estrogen. Her pituitary gland increases production of other hormones. These hormonal changes are responsible for the symptoms commonly associated with the menopause, which include sudden flushing and severe sweating (hot flashes), insomnia, dryness of the skin and of the vagina, depression, irritability, and fatigue.

A positive approach to menopause
Some women dread menopause because they think it means the onset of uncomfortable symptoms. However, many women experience a new feeling of freedom and vitality because they no longer need to cope with menstruation or worry about becoming pregnant.

Osteoporosis

Both men and women lose bone mass and strength steadily after age 35 as part of the natural aging process. However, for women, the rate of bone loss rapidly accelerates at the time of menopause because of the effects of altered hormone production. Osteoporosis, a condition that leaves the bones more porous, more fragile, and more susceptible to fracture, affects about one third of all postmenopausal women in the US, many of whom do not experience any symptoms. Lost bone tissue cannot be easily replaced, but you can minimize further bone loss. Include calcium (found in milk and milk products and green leafy vegetables) in your diet, and exercise regularly. Smoking and alcohol and caffeine consumption are among the factors that reduce bone density. Hormone replacement therapy can compensate for reduced estrogen production.

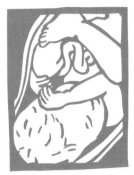

MONITOR YOUR PREGNANCY

FOR A BABY TO BE HEALTHY, the father's sperm and the mother's egg must be normal and the fetus must be protected from harm. By taking steps to ensure that you and your partner are as healthy as possible before conception and by being alert to signs of sickness during pregnancy and breast-feeding, you will give yourself and your baby the best possible chance of good health.

FACTORS TO DISCUSS WITH YOUR DOCTOR BEFORE CONCEPTION

◆ **Medication** Talk about any drugs that you or your partner are taking or planning to take; some drugs could have harmful effects on the developing fetus. If you are taking an oral contraceptive, your doctor may suggest that you switch to another method of contraception before you stop using contraceptives altogether.

◆ **Immunization** Check with your doctor or check your immunization records to verify that you are immune to rubella (German measles). If you were to contract the disease during pregnancy, the fetus could be harmed.

◆ **Medical disorders** If you have a condition such as diabetes, epilepsy, or heart disease, discuss the implications for you and the fetus.

A number of factors affecting the health of parents-to-be may increase health risks to the fetus.

HEALTH CONCERNS BEFORE CONCEPTION

It is ideal to begin thinking seriously about your health 3 to 6 months before you begin trying to conceive.

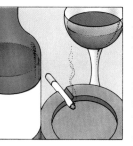

Smoking, alcohol consumption, and other drug use Smoking, alcohol consumption, or the use of other drugs such as marijuana and cocaine can harm a fetus. The best advice for you and your partner is to give up any drugs you use.

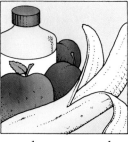

Dietary factors When you are pregnant, remember that the fetus's tissues are formed by your body's use of the foods you eat. To supplement your healthy diet, your doctor may prescribe vitamins and iron to ensure that the fetus has what it needs to develop normally.

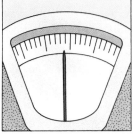

Weight Being overweight or underweight can adversely affect both the pregnant woman and the fetus. It is helpful to ensure that your weight falls within an appropriate range before you conceive.

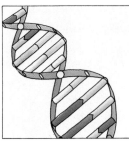

Genetic disorders Couples who have a family history of genetic diseases, such as Tay-Sachs disease, sickle cell trait, or hemophilia, are advised to obtain genetic counseling to learn their risk of having affected children. Screening can detect the presence of some gene defects.

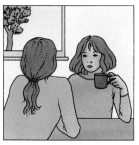

Choosing your doctor It is important to choose an obstetrician you trust. Get recommendations from friends and visit local hospitals to see their facilities. When you talk to your doctor, ask questions freely and volunteer information about yourself.

CONFIRMING THE PREGNANCY

The most common sign of pregnancy is missing your menstrual period. However, a number of physical changes may alert you to the possibility of pregnancy. In the first few weeks of pregnancy, your breasts usually start to feel fuller, your nipples enlarge, and the veins on your breasts become more prominent. You may urinate more frequently and find that vaginal secretions increase. Many women experience nausea (so-called morning sickness) between about the sixth and the 14th week.

PROFESSIONAL PREGNANCY TESTING

Your doctor may use the following techniques.

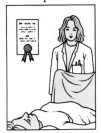

♦ **Physical examination** Your doctor may perform an internal (vaginal) examination to evaluate the size of your uterus. He or she may also look for changes in your cervix and breasts.

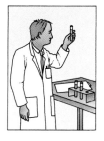

♦ **Testing urine for human chorionic gonadotropin (HCG)** After a physical examination, a sample of urine is sent to the laboratory to confirm the presence of HCG.

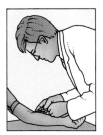

♦ **Blood testing** Blood tests for pregnancy are highly accurate and are often used if there is reason to question the result of the urine test. Blood tests are used to confirm tubal or other abnormal pregnancies.

Home pregnancy testing

During pregnancy, a woman's body produces a hormone called human chorionic gonadotropin (sometimes abbreviated HCG). Pregnancy test kits can now detect HCG quite shortly after you miss your period. Many home testing kits claim to be 99 percent accurate if used correctly. At best, this means you have a 1 percent chance of obtaining a false result. If you obtain a positive result, consult your doctor for further confirmation. If you obtain a negative result, repeat the home test 1 week later if your period has not begun. Talk to your doctor if your test result remains negative but you still have not had a period.

To reduce the possibility of obtaining a false result, it is advisable to wait until your period is at least 2 weeks late before doing a home test. Some women who are especially eager to conceive may experience a disruption in their menstrual cycle because of anxiety.

How do home testing kits work?
Home pregnancy testing kits, such as the one illustrated below, usually require you to combine a sample of urine (obtained first thing in the morning) with test chemicals. Then you insert a test stick into the liquid. The stick is coated with chemicals that react with the pregnancy hormone human chorionic gonadotropin (HCG). If your urine contains HCG, the stick changes color when dipped in a special solution to indicate a positive result. The exact procedure for performing the test varies among brands, so be certain you follow the manufacturer's instructions precisely.

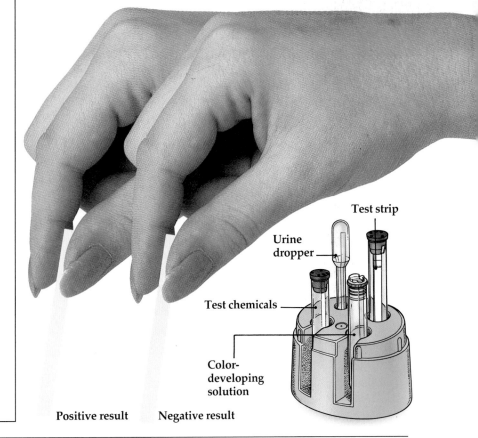

Test strip

Urine dropper

Test chemicals

Color-developing solution

Positive result   **Negative result**

PRENATAL CARE

To ensure that you remain healthy throughout pregnancy, and that the fetus develops normally, regular medical care is essential. As soon as your pregnancy is confirmed, talk to your doctor about prenatal care. Your doctor will schedule several examinations and tests – including weight checkups, blood pressure measurements, and blood and urine tests. If there is uncertainty about the age of the fetus or if other questions arise about the fetus's health or position in the uterus, your doctor may want to perform ultrasound scanning.

By 3 weeks after conception (5 weeks after the last period), ultrasound can distinguish ectopic (i.e., tubal) pregnancies from normal pregnancies. By 5 weeks after conception (7 weeks after the last period), ultrasound can determine the number of fetuses and whether a fetus is alive and growing. Ultrasound is used to detect some fetal abnormalities and is also used as a guide for further diagnostic tests such as chorionic villus sampling or amniocentesis. These procedures also test for fetal abnormalities.

Taking care of yourself

During pregnancy, your daily energy requirements increase by about 300 kilocalories. You need more protein and vitamins and almost twice as much calcium as normal. A balanced diet should supply you with sufficient quantities. Many doctors prescribe folic acid and iron supplements for pregnant women. Stop smoking and drinking alcohol and avoid all drugs unless your doctor prescribes them. Women who are taking any medication when they get pregnant should notify their doctors immediately because the medication may be discontinued.

Keeping a "kick chart"
Your doctor may encourage you to keep a "kick chart" to monitor the fetus's movements inside your uterus, which you can feel by about the 20th week. Report any decrease in the number of kicks.

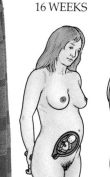

16 WEEKS	22 WEEKS	28 WEEKS	34 WEEKS	40 WEEKS

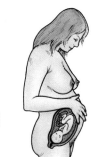

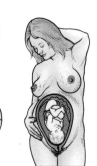

MINOR HEALTH PROBLEMS

Pregnant women may experience health problems such as backache, breathlessness, constipation, hemorrhoids, leg cramps, heartburn, faintness, increased skin pigmentation, varicose veins, greater urinary frequency, and vaginal yeast infections. Many of these problems clear up once the baby is born. If your symptoms become troublesome, talk to your doctor about them.

WARNING

The following warning signs should be reported to your doctor immediately:

♦ Vaginal bleeding
♦ Excessive or sudden swelling of the ankles, face, and hands
♦ Severe vomiting
♦ Severe pain in the abdomen
♦ Fever
♦ Severe persistent headache
♦ Chest pain and breathlessness

BREAST-FEEDING

While you are breast-feeding your baby, you may feel hungrier and thirstier than usual. As your baby grows, your daily energy requirements will increase by about 500 kilocalories. The quality of the breast milk you produce is directly related to the quality of your diet. Eating a well-balanced variety of foods is more important than ever when you are breast-feeding. Too much caffeine may make your baby irritable, so try to reduce your intake. Other drugs may also enter the breast milk and affect your baby. Alcohol or barbiturates, for example, can cause drowsiness, and laxatives can cause diarrhea. Oral contraceptives pass through the breast milk, and most doctors recommend that nursing women avoid them. If an oral contraceptive is necessary, progestogen-only contraceptives are considered safe after about 6 weeks. Always check with your doctor before taking any drugs.

BREAST-FEEDING PROBLEMS

Painful fullness of the breasts
If your breasts feel hard and painfully full you need to express the surplus milk.

Breast inflammation
Talk to your doctor if your breasts feel painful and are inflamed on the surface. You may have contracted a breast infection.

Abnormal-looking or blood-stained milk
Breast milk that contains blood or is discolored may indicate infection. Call your doctor.

Breast lumps
Consult your doctor if you discover a lump or persistent swelling in your breast.

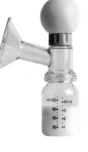

Breast pumps
You can express milk by hand or with a breast pump. Expressing relieves any accumulation of breast milk, and you can freeze the milk so that your baby can be bottle-fed when you are away.

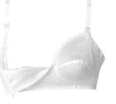

Nursing bras
A nursing bra should provide firm support. Some bras, such as the one pictured above, are designed with cups that open separately so you can feed your baby easily.

Sore nipples
Soreness of the nipples is a common problem for breast-feeding women. It may be relieved by using an emollient cream.

Cracked nipples
If sore nipples are not treated, painful cracks may develop, making the breasts more vulnerable to infection.

MONITOR YOUR PREGNANCY

Q How often do miscarriages occur, and can you explain what causes them?

A Possibly as many as one in three pregnancies ends in a miscarriage. However, the incidence is difficult to determine because an early miscarriage may manifest itself as a heavy period. About half of all miscarriages occur because the fetus is abnormal. Other causes include infections, chronic illness, drug use, autoimmune reactions, and abnormalities of the uterus or cervix. Lifting, carrying, exercise, or intercourse do not usually cause miscarriage.

Q I like to drink some form of alcoholic beverage almost every day. Will I have to give up alcohol altogether during pregnancy?

A Drinking alcohol can result in fetal alcohol syndrome, a condition in which the baby's growth is stunted and the baby is physically abnormal and mentally retarded. Even a single "binge" of heavy drinking may be harmful. No one knows exactly what the safe limit is, so doctors advise against drinking any alcohol during pregnancy.

Q Can sexual intercourse be harmful at any stage of pregnancy?

A There is no evidence that sexual intercourse during a normal pregnancy is harmful. However, if you have had a previous miscarriage, or have had any bleeding during the early stages of pregnancy, your doctor may recommend that you not have intercourse during the first 14 weeks.

CHAPTER THREE

MONITOR YOUR MENTAL AND EMOTIONAL HEALTH

INTRODUCTION

KNOW YOURSELF

SIGNS OF
MENTAL PROBLEMS

WHAT KIND OF PERSON are you? Do you think of yourself as bright, assertive, and stable, brimming with self-confidence and happiness? Or are you only rarely sure of yourself? Perhaps you have difficulty contemplating your level of self-fulfillment and your emotional welfare. But these are important areas, like physical health, that need our attention if we wish to maximize our overall well-being and happiness.

While our temperament and reactions to stress are to some extent determined by genetic factors, we can achieve a great deal in these areas through our own initiative, sometimes with professional help as well. Counseling, behavior modification, or psychoanalytic therapy, for example, have helped many people resolve serious mental or emotional difficulties, work through troubling

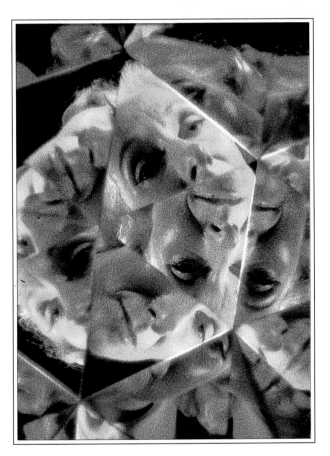

life crises, or simply realize their potential more fully. But the key is self-awareness. We must first recognize and admit to difficulties before we can attempt constructive methods of dealing with them. Today, unlike in the past, mental health professionals and the public alike accept the fact that personality difficulties and emotional stress affect virtually all of us to some degree. It is how we adapt to and

cope with these difficulties that determines our ultimate happiness. We all have problems at certain times in our lives that may respond to thoughtful self-analysis or outside help. Even reasonably well-adjusted people can enhance their effectiveness and happiness by gaining insight into their emotional lives and by taking advantage of some of the psychological knowledge and techniques that are available today. The importance of monitoring our mental and emotional health is threefold. First, it offers the opportunity to change our outlook and lifestyle for the better and to cope more effectively with emotional problems such as depression, anxiety, guilt, or grief. Second, it may lead to recognition of a serious mental problem that requires professional treatment. Third, it may even improve our physical health.

This chapter describes some of the methods that mental health professionals use for understanding personality, mental ability, emotional stability, and general functioning. We give you some indication as to when professional help is called for. Perhaps the most important point to keep in mind is that, if emotional difficulties significantly interfere with your well-being, effective treatment is available.

KNOW YOURSELF

I N ORDER TO RECOGNIZE that psychological or emotional problems are developing it is helpful first to understand your usual personality traits and state of mind. Against this background of self-awareness, you can better recognize how you respond to stress and when you may need professional help or other treatment.

In this section, we offer an idea of how mental health professionals assess personality types. We describe some of the signs that may indicate mental or emotional problems. You will also learn how your general mental ability and, more specifically, your memory may be affected by mood, level of stress, and a variety of disorders.

PERSONALITY

The study of personality and how it develops has fascinated researchers for many years. Some theories, such as the well-known work of Sigmund Freud, focus on childhood and successful passage through the emotional stages we go through before the age of 5. Other influential theories, including those of Carl Jung, maintain that personality develops over the course of a lifetime. An individual's personality and how he or she copes with stress may contribute to the development of some diseases, such as coronary heart disease, hypertension, and migraine headache. However, there is also significant genetic predisposition toward these conditions.

Efforts to describe personality types are always controversial. Most people do not fall exclusively into any single group, but display traits from one or more groups to some degree. Your personality type does not determine whether you are mentally healthy. Each of us has some psychological conflicts. Your personality traits are a problem only if they interfere substantially with your relationships with others, your profession,

PERSONALITY ASSESSMENT

One well-known personality assessment tool uses four scales, shown here, to describe a person's perceptions and preferences. From your responses to a written questionnaire, a psychologist would derive a score on each scale, then interpret the results to help guide you in important areas of your life.

PREFERENCE SCALES

Extroversion-Introversion (EI)
The EI index reflects whether you are oriented primarily toward the outer world (E) or toward the inner world of ideas (I).

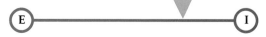

Sensing-Intuition (SN)
The SN index describes an interest in perceiving the objects, events, and details of the present moment (S) or the possibilities, abstractions, and insights of the future (N).

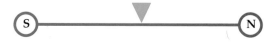

Thinking-Feeling (TF)
The TF index describes a preference for making decisions by using objective and logical analysis (T) or by weighing the relative person-centered values (F).

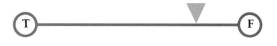

Judging-Perceiving (JP)
The JP index describes your preference for organizing and controlling events (J) or for observing and understanding these events (P).

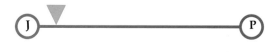

or other important aspects of your life, or if they contribute to the development of unhealthy habits such as overeating or abuse of alcohol.

Psychological testing

Psychological tests provide a fairly objective picture of your intelligence, your personality, and how you function emotionally. The results of these tests can help guide diagnosis and treatment of mental disorders. Mental health professionals may use personality tests to help individuals recognize emotional problems and conflicts that may be adversely affecting their lives.

Standardized scales used to score the tests are based on data from control groups to ensure that the test is valid (that it measures what it is intended to measure) and is reliable (produces consistent results). One of the most commonly used personality tests is the Minnesota Multiphasic Personality In-

ventory. When you take the test, you respond to 550 true/false questions such as "I worry about sex matters," "I believe I am being plotted against," or "I sometimes tease animals." The test is numerically scored and statistically analyzed. Accurate interpretation of your score is complex, involving some understanding of the socioeconomic and educational influences in your life. Recent evidence suggests that cultural factors such as religion and race also may affect your responses.

Other personality tests are projective – that is, you assign meaning to some stimulus (a picture, an inkblot, or an incomplete sentence) according to your own inner needs, conflicts, and defenses. There are no right or wrong answers. Interpretation of the results requires extensive experience, but a professional can gain insight into different levels of mental functioning through the use of projective tests.

THE INKBLOT TEST

One of the most famous projective personality tests is the Rorschach inkblot test. Developed in 1910, it is still useful today. You are asked to say what you "see" in each of a standard set of inkblots. The test is designed to help reveal unconscious thought and association patterns. The results must be interpreted by a psychologist.

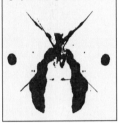

HOW A PSYCHOLOGIST USES PERSONALITY ASSESSMENT

A mental health professional can interpret your responses to a personality test to assist you in self-exploration and decision-making.

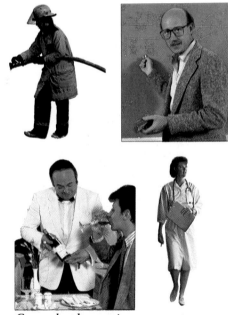

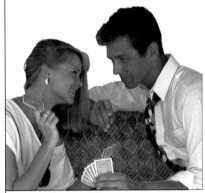

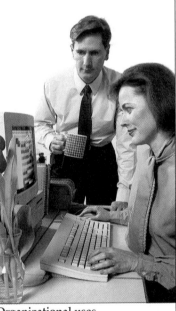

Personal counseling
With guidance you can learn to build on your strengths, better understand similarities and differences between yourself and others, and improve the quality of your personal relationships and interactions.

Career development
A psychologist may use the assessment to help you identify the work environment to which you are best suited and to relate career performance, opportunities, and demands to your preferences.

Organizational uses
Within an organization, professional personality testing can help improve teamwork and communication among colleagues, develop management style, and resolve conflicts.

WHAT IS YOUR EMOTIONAL ATTITUDE?

You may be interested in testing yourself on a questionnaire that is similar in some respects to psychological tests used by mental health professionals. It takes a well-trained psychologist to accurately evaluate the results of such a test. This test simply provides you with a sampling of ways to evaluate how you are doing emotionally in the areas of anxiety, depression, and self-esteem. We probably all have been anxious, depressed, or full of self-doubt at one time or another. Your scores on this test will not indicate whether you have an emotional problem that interferes significantly with your life. Keep in mind that these questions – like those in any do-it-yourself psychological quiz – are very general. You should be cautious about drawing any firm conclusions about your emotional status from such questions. If your responses or your scores raise any troubling questions for you, you may want to discuss them with a mental health professional. Answer "yes" or "no" to each question and don't leave any questions unanswered. Then total your scores according to the instructions and read the interpretations given on page 74.

	ANXIETY	DEPRESSION	SELF-ESTEEM
1	Do you worry unreasonably over things that don't really matter?	Do things often seem hopeless to you?	Are you fairly sure of yourself most of the time?
2	If you have made a social mistake can you easily forget it?	Do you smile and laugh more than most people?	Do you often think of yourself as a failure?
3	Do you feel anxious about something or somebody nearly all the time?	Have you often felt listless and tired for no clear reason?	Are you happy with your physical appearance?
4	Do you relax easily when you are sitting down?	Are you bothered a lot by noise?	Do you often wish you were someone else?
5	Do you tend to get "rattled" if things don't go according to plan?	Do you feel that you often get a raw deal in life?	Would you be troubled by feelings of inadequacy if you had to make a speech?
6	Would you stay cool and collected in the face of danger?	Do you often feel that people don't care what happens to you?	Do you often feel ashamed of things you have done?
7	Do you sometimes feel you have so many problems that you'll never overcome them?	Do you suffer a lot from loneliness?	Do you think you do things as well as most people?
8	As a child, were you afraid of the dark?	Do you find much happiness in life?	Do you suffer from feelings of inferiority?
9	Do you blush more than most people?	Do you often feel you don't care what happens to you?	Do some members of your family make you feel you are not good enough for them?
10	Would you say that you seldom lose sleep over your worries?	Are you in good spirits most of the time?	Do you have a great deal of confidence in the correctness of your decisions?
11	Are you usually calm and easygoing?	Do you often feel "just terrible" without good reason?	Does it seem to you that photographs never do you justice?

12	Are you easily startled by someone appearing unexpectedly?	Does your future look bright to you?	Are there a lot of things about yourself that you would change if you could?
13	Do you find it impossible to sit still without fidgeting?	Have you ever wished you were dead?	Do you feel you have nothing to be proud of?
14	Do you worry regularly over money matters?	Do you seem to have more than your share of bad luck?	Do you think your personality is attractive to the opposite sex?
15	Generally speaking, are you a nervous person?	In general, would you say you are satisfied with your life?	Does it sometimes seem that you can never do anything right?
16	Have you ever felt you needed to take tranquilizers?	Do you often feel down in the dumps?	Are you often reticent because you think other people will not like you?
17	Are you inclined to get worked up over nothing?	Do you wake up in the morning feeling vigorous and "ready to go"?	Do you usually feel able to accomplish the things you want?
18	Do you worry too long over a humiliating experience?	Would you say you are leading a useful and rewarding life?	Do you often not give your opinion because you think people will criticize you or laugh at you?
19	Would you describe yourself as a self-conscious person?	Is there at least one person in the world who really loves you?	Do you often question your worth as a person?
20	Do you worry about things that you think might happen?	Would you be reluctant to bring a child into the world the way things are today?	Does everyone else seem more successful in life than you?
21	Can you drop off to sleep easily at night?	Have you been generally successful in achieving your goals in life?	Would you say you have a high opinion of yourself?
22	Are you easily embarrassed in social situations?	Do you often get the feeling that you are just not a part of things?	Are there parts of your body that you try to disguise by clothing because you think they are unattractive?
23	Do you often wake up in a sweat after having a nightmare?	Is your sleep fitful and disturbed?	Do you think you are generally popular with other people?
24	Does your voice get shaky when you are talking to someone you want to impress?	Are you inclined to feel lonely even when you are with other people?	Did you do very well at school?
25	Do you become tense when you think about your problems?	Do you have a sense of inner calm and contentment?	Are you reluctant to visit doctors because you don't want to waste their time?
26	Are you more prone to anxiety than most of your friends?	Do you feel cheated when you look back on the things that have happened to you?	Do people regard you as useful to have around?
27	Do you tremble and perspire if faced with a difficult task?	Are you about as happy as the next person?	Do you often have doubts about your sexual ability?
28	Do you often feel restless, as though you want something but don't really know what?	Does it seem to you other people always get the breaks?	Do you find it difficult to do things in a way that generates approval from others?
29	Are you afraid of things and people that you know would not really hurt you?	Are you often overwhelmed with sadness?	Do you find that people try to avoid your company because they find you boring?
30	Does life often seem to be a strain for you?	Has it been a long time since you last felt on top of the world?	Do you get very upset if someone criticizes you?

SCORING AND INTERPRETING THE EMOTIONAL ATTITUDE TEST

This test is designed so that the average person usually scores toward the middle of each range (from 10 to 20). If you score 20 or higher on the anxiety or depression sections or below 10 on the self-esteem section, you might want to consider seeking advice from a mental health professional.

ANXIETY

Give yourself one point for each "yes" you answered to questions 1, 3, 5, 7, 8, 9, 12, 13, 14, 15, 16, 17, 18, 19, 20, 22, 23, 24, 25, 26, 27, 28, 29, and 30 and each "no" you answered to questions 2, 4, 6, 10, 11, and 21. This will give you an "anxiety score."

Anxiety is an emotional state that reflects inner or psychological fears. An anxious person often has a sense of impending doom. Symptoms such as compulsions, phobias, or defense mechanisms employed to combat anxiety may develop in people who score 20 or higher. Panic attacks (see page 80) are outbreaks of extreme anxiety that defense mechanisms can no longer contain.

DEPRESSION

Give yourself one point for each "yes" you answered to questions 1, 3, 4, 5, 6, 7, 9, 11, 13, 14, 16, 20, 22, 23, 24, 26, 28, 29, and 30 and each "no" you answered to questions 2, 8, 10, 12, 15, 17, 18, 19, 21, 25, and 27. This will give you a "depression score."

Depression is an emotional reaction of sadness or despair. A depressed person tends to feel pessimistic, hopeless, and indifferent. A person normally experiences these feelings in reaction to loss. High scorers on this scale (those who score 20 or higher) are nearly always unhappy and may tend toward a depressive disorder for which professional treatment is needed (see page 79).

SELF-ESTEEM

Give yourself one point for each "yes" you answered to questions 1, 3, 7, 10, 14, 17, 21, 23, 24, and 26 and each "no" to questions 2,4, 5, 6, 8, 9, 11, 12, 13, 15, 16, 18, 19, 20, 22, 25, 27, 28, 29, and 30. This will give you a "self-esteem score."

Psychological testing, in addition to analyzing emotions, can also measure psychological attitudes (for instance, your self-image as measured by your self-esteem). High scorers in this category (those who score 20 or higher) have confidence in themselves and their abilities. Low scorers (those who score less than 10) have a very low opinion of themselves that is unjustified and self-defeating.

The IQ test
One example of a performance test is shown below. You would be asked to put the puzzle together and would be given a score according to your accuracy and the length of time you took.

GENERAL MENTAL ABILITY

How well you are able to perform any mental task varies according to the external situation, your mood or frame of mind, and your level of motivation. Although mental ability does not necessarily deteriorate with age, an older person may learn new material more slowly and experience some memory impairment. At any age, a psycho-logical problem such as depression or anxiety can interfere with concentration and memory. If your concentration, general alertness, or mental responses are causing you persistent problems that interfere with your daily functioning, you may benefit from professional help.

A psychologist evaluating your range of mental functions would use psychological tests, including an IQ (intelligence quotient) test. An IQ test measures your present ability, not your future potential. No intelligence test is free of cultural bias. One of the widely used IQ tests is the Wechsler Adult Intelligence Scale. It has two sections – a verbal portion that tests language skills, vocabulary, general knowledge, reasoning, and memory, and a performance portion that tests visual/spatial and perceptual abilities. The IQ test is designed so that the majority of people who take the test score between 80 and 120.

CASE HISTORY
PERFORMANCE PROBLEMS

NICK WAS PASSED OVER for the third time for a promotion in favor of less able colleagues. His social life was also not satisfying. He had not felt confident enough to ask a woman for a date in 6 months. Nick began to feel depressed and had frequent headaches. His repeated absence from work ultimately caused him to be fired. At this point an old friend suggested that he seek professional help.

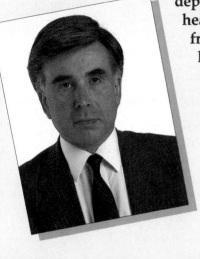

PERSONAL DETAILS
Name Nick Zeller
Age 45
Occupation Telephone company dispatcher
Family Both parents are well. Nick has an older brother who is married and lives in another city.

MEDICAL BACKGROUND
Nick has had no major medical problems but tends to get headaches, colds, and other minor infections more than most people.

THE CONSULTATION
At first, Nick tells the doctor that he is worried about his recurrent headaches. However, the doctor soon realizes that this concern is not the real reason for Nick's visit. As she questions Nick more closely, she discovers that Nick is desperately unhappy because of his professional and social problems. The doctor refers Nick to a psychiatrist.

THE CONSULTATION WITH THE PSYCHIATRIST
During several interviews with the psychiatrist, Nick reveals that at work he has always felt his skills were not recognized or appreciated. When the psychiatrist asks why he has never complained to his supervisor, Nick admits that he has been afraid that he might not be able to compete at a higher managerial level. In response to questions about his family, Nick recalls that his older brother was an excellent student. No matter how hard Nick tried, his parents always boasted about his brother's achievements but not about his. As he discusses his social life, he reveals that he always fears women will think he has not been successful for someone his age.

THE DIAGNOSIS
The psychiatrist concludes that Nick's problems are due to EMOTIONAL CONFLICTS AND LOW SELF-ESTEEM. Nick's early experiences with his family caused him to learn a negative, self-defeating pattern of thoughts and behavior. His lack of assertiveness at work and in social situations set up a vicious circle that caused him to behave in an even more timid and self-effacing way.

THE TREATMENT
The psychiatrist establishes a supportive, encouraging relationship with Nick, which enables Nick to express his fears of rejection at work and with women. The psychiatrist helps him see how his parents' favored treatment of his brother made him feel that he lacked attractive qualities of his own.

THE OUTCOME
Therapy helps Nick understand his fears and work through them. At his weekly sessions, Nick begins to learn positive ways to view himself and his experiences. He interviews for jobs and gets a good opportunity. He is looking forward to meeting women through his new work.

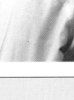

Learning about himself
Nick's sessions with the psychiatrist help him turn negative, self-defeating thoughts and behavior into a more productive outlook.

MEMORY

About 100 billion neurons (nerve cells) in your brain are involved in forming memories, essential components of learning. When you receive new information, electrochemical impulses pass through neurons and stimulate the development of new neural connections. Storage is the key to a good memory. Relating new information to something you already know creates more connections and increases your storage power. Your mood affects your ability to store and recall information. When you are in a happy mood, you remember what you learn better and you can better recall what you have learned previously. Too much stress adversely affects both short-term and long-term memory. The increase in epinephrine (a hormone that results from stress) can enhance learning but, if the stress is too great or lasts too long, learning is inhibited. Your short-term, or "working," memory is particularly impaired by emotional stress.

Brain injuries and diseases can result in a severe degree of memory loss. The inability to remember the events immediately preceding a blow to the head (known as retrograde amnesia) is well-known. Chronic alcoholism can lead to a condition that results in severe loss of short-term memory, without significantly affecting long-term memory. A greater impairment of short-term memory may also be apparent in conditions such as Alzheimer's disease, other forms of dementia, and stroke. It should be kept in mind, however, that depression or anxiety can impair memory to a significant extent even though no organic brain damage has occurred.

The mystery of Alzheimer's disease
The photograph of brain tissue below reveals the presence of an amyloid plaque. This deposit, composed of protein, starch, and other substances, is one of the characteristics of Alzheimer's disease. Although the cause of the disease is still unknown, a poor memory when you are young does not indicate an increased risk of the disease.

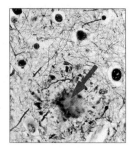

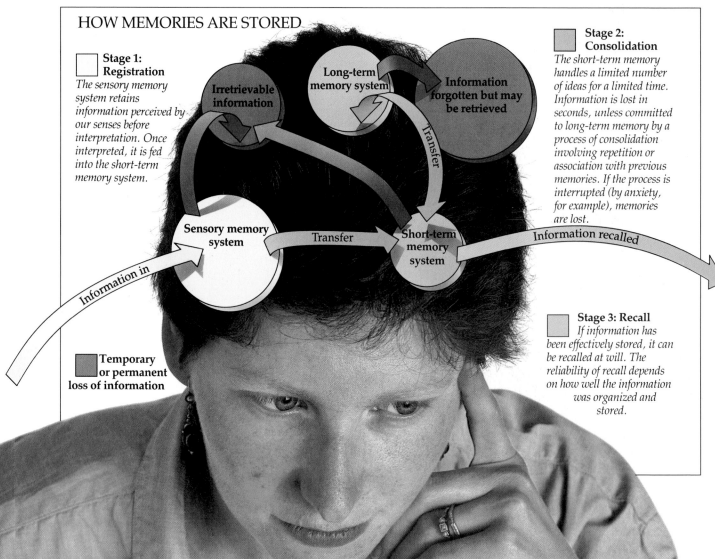

HOW MEMORIES ARE STORED

Stage 1: Registration
The sensory memory system retains information perceived by our senses before interpretation. Once interpreted, it is fed into the short-term memory system.

Stage 2: Consolidation
The short-term memory handles a limited number of ideas for a limited time. Information is lost in seconds, unless committed to long-term memory by a process of consolidation involving repetition or association with previous memories. If the process is interrupted (by anxiety, for example), memories are lost.

Stage 3: Recall
If information has been effectively stored, it can be recalled at will. The reliability of recall depends on how well the information was organized and stored.

Irretrievable information

Long-term memory system

Information forgotten but may be retrieved

Sensory memory system

Short-term memory system

Information in

Transfer

Transfer

Information recalled

Temporary or permanent loss of information

TEST YOUR SHORT-TERM MEMORY

Doctors and psychologists use a variety of tests to assess memory and intellectual function. Some tests are long and standardized (including the Wechsler Adult Intelligence Scales) while others are simple tests that can be conducted in the office. Tests such as those outlined below may be used for self-testing of short-term memory, but they cannot stand as definitive tests unless conducted and assessed by a trained professional. However, if you find these exercises particularly difficult, you may have some problem with your short-term memory that you might want to discuss with your doctor.

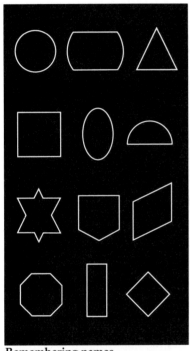

Reproducing shapes
Study the shapes on the dark background at left for exactly 2 minutes and then cover them up. See how many you can reproduce on a piece of blank paper. The order in which you reproduce them is not important. The average person remembers about half the shapes.

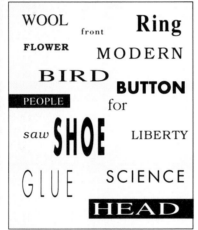

Remembering names
Look at the faces of the people shown below for 1 minute and try to memorize their names. Close this book and do something else for half an hour. Then turn immediately to the appendix on page 141 without looking again at the pictures and see how many of the faces you can name. If you remember fewer than half, you may have a problem with short-term memory.

Recalling words
Study the words above for exactly 2 minutes, writing them down in any order on a blank piece of paper if you think that will help you remember them. Close this book and write down as many of the words as you can remember on a fresh piece of paper. The average person remembers about half the words.

Memorizing pairs of colors
Starting from the top, memorize the colors of the pairs of rectangles above. Spend about 10 seconds on each pair and cover up the surrounding pairs with two pieces of paper as you do so. Now cover up the entire right-hand column and work down the left-hand column, exposing only one rectangle at a time. Try to recall the corresponding right-hand color. Check each answer as you go but cover up the rectangles once you have checked. Do something else for about half an hour. Then repeat the test, trying to recall the colors of the pairs again. After doing the test a few times, you should be able to remember all the color pairs.

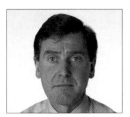

Max

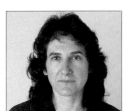

Alice

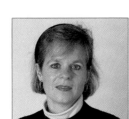

Diane

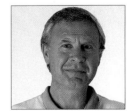

Ted

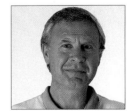

Martha

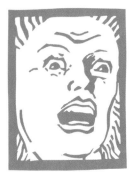

SIGNS OF MENTAL PROBLEMS

WE ALL HAVE TIMES when we feel worried, frustrated, or dejected. No one feels happy all the time. When we have problems, often just talking to someone close can help. But sometimes depression, anxiety, or other disturbing feelings will not go away, and professional help may be needed.

SIGNS OF MENTAL ILLNESS

The American Psychiatric Association has compiled a list of signs that could indicate that a person has a mental illness. The warning signs are described here.

Mental and emotional disturbances can affect your mood, your behavior, your level of functioning, and your physical health. Prolonged or severe emotional stress can seriously affect many areas of your life, such as your work and your relationships with your family or friends. In some cases, it may be vital that you or someone you know seek professional treatment to identify, fully understand, and work through the problem.

WHAT ARE THE COMMON MENTAL PROBLEMS?

Depression and anxiety are the most common psychiatric illnesses affecting Americans. About 10 to 15 percent of Americans experience some form of depressive illness (characterized by chronic or prolonged feelings of sadness or hopelessness) at some time in their lives.

Strange or grandiose ideas
Delusions that a person has special powers or knowledge or has a special relationship with a deity or famous person.

Prolonged depression and apathy
Lack of interest in anything; the feeling that life is pointless and an unrelenting sequence of worry and unhappiness.

Excessive anger, hostility, or violent behavior
Extreme instability of mood or recurrent outbursts of rage, grossly out of proportion to the situation.

Abuse of alcohol or other drugs
Inability to control one's use of alcohol or use of other drugs (legal or illegal).

Anxiety disorders, characterized by a state of fear, affect about 4 percent of the population. There is often overlap between these two disorders and people may have symptoms of both.

Depression

People often feel low for brief periods, especially when they are experiencing difficult circumstances. This is not a depression. A true depressive illness seriously affects a person's behavior and physical state. The rate of reported depression has increased in recent years. A 1989 study showed that 58 percent of Americans born after 1955 have reported a case of depression. The rising rate may reflect greater willingness to seek help for mental disorders. Depression is one of the most treatable forms of psychiatric illness. However, it is sometimes not diagnosed because patients have difficulty describing symptoms and doctors have difficulty interpreting them. A depressed person may suffer from anxiety, irritability, and loss of sexual interest and may withdraw from social contact and abandon leisure interests. If the person also has sleep problems and losses of appetite, weight, and concentration, he or she quite probably is suffering from a severe depression. A visit to a doctor is called for.

Depression may be triggered by major changes in your life, such as moving, having a baby, or the death of someone close (see SCALE OF LIFE EVENTS on page 91). Some psychiatrists view depression as an inherited trait or a chemical imbalance. Others regard depression as having an emotional origin, resulting from life experiences and losses.

PHYSICAL SYMPTOMS OF ANXIETY

A person who has an anxiety disorder may experience any of these symptoms:

♦ Sweating
♦ Palpitations
♦ Difficulty breathing
♦ Trembling
♦ Headaches and muscular aches
♦ Dizziness
♦ Tension
♦ Fatigue
♦ Numbness or tingling
♦ Upset stomach
♦ Diarrhea
♦ Lump in the throat
♦ Weight loss

Excessive anxieties
An irrational terror that comes on suddenly (panic attack) or a nagging sense of apprehension (generalized anxiety).

Marked personality change
For example, a striking increase in fatigue and irritability or strange or inappropriate behavior.

Marked changes in eating or sleeping patterns
Eating problems that take the form of starvation (anorexia nervosa), bulimia (binge-purge syndrome), overeating, or other extreme dietary patterns. A person may have difficulty sleeping or may sleep all the time.

Inability to cope
Difficulty coping with problems and daily activities at work or at home. The person may have trouble making friends, keeping a job, or taking care of his or her family responsibilities.

Anxiety disorders

Within certain limits, anxiety is healthy and beneficial. We all need to be stimulated, to strive for goals, and to adapt to change. Anxiety, or fear, is designed to protect us from danger. When anxiety occurs in response to psychological pressures out of proportion to the situation, it may disrupt thought and activity. An extreme form of anxiety disorder is a panic attack, a spontaneous, intense outbreak of anxiety. In some people, panic attacks occur without apparent reason. When they are associated with one particular object or situation, they are known as phobias. Phobias, which affect from 5 to 12 percent of the population, most often appear in response to such things as insects, animals, and heights.

Hand-washing compulsion
This is one of the most common obsessive-compulsive disorders. The individual worries about infection and may spend hours washing his or her hands, sometimes until the skin is raw and bleeding. The unconscious psychological issue may be unrelated to infection.

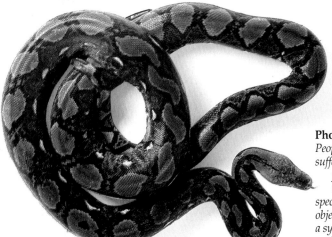

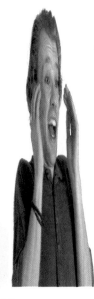

Phobias
People with a phobia suffer from an irrational fear of a specific object (such as a snake) or a specific situation. The object or situation is only a symbol of the underlying emotional conflict, which is likely to concern other people.

Panic attacks
Panic attacks are frightening episodes in which the victim is overcome with terror and suffers from a variety of symptoms that may include sweating, palpitations, hot or cold flashes, feelings of unreality, choking or smothering sensations, difficulty breathing, faintness, tingling, and fear of going crazy.

Obsessive-compulsive behavior is a more rare form of anxiety. Obsessions are repeated, unwanted thoughts; compulsions are behaviors performed for no reason other than to allay anxiety. They are rituals used to ward off unconscious emotional conflicts that a person fears will be overwhelming if expressed consciously. Many people exhibit some degree of obsessive-compulsive behavior, such as checking and rechecking whether doors are locked. In this instance, the obsessive thought is doubt and the compulsive behavior is the constant checking. Such behavior becomes a problem only if it starts to take up so much time that it interferes with a person's daily living.

Anxiety does not always manifest itself in such a sudden and dramatic way. It may take the form of a constant sense of apprehension (free-floating anxiety) combined with various symptoms throughout the body (see page 79).

Agoraphobia
People with this particularly disabling phobia are afraid to be alone in public or crowded places. They avoid going out in public for fear of having a panic attack and eventually may become completely housebound. Treatment with psychotherapy and antidepressants is usually successful in helping victims resolve their underlying unconscious emotional conflicts.

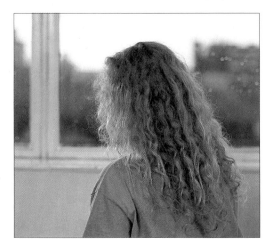

DIARY OF A DEPRESSION

Below are some selected examples of entries in a diary kept by David, a 47-year-old computer programmer who lives with his wife Beth and their three children. These entries illustrate the progression of David's depressive illness, the effects it had on his attitude and performance, the fact that neither his wife nor his doctor recognized his problem until it had become severe, and David's first steps toward recovery. In such a case, the eventual diagnosis of depression will probably make it easier to prevent or control any future episodes with medical help and reassurance that the depression will lift. David, his family, and his doctor will also be better prepared to recognize symptoms of a developing depression.

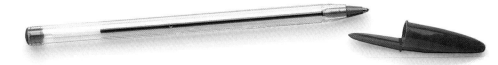

February 3
It seems like a long time since I really enjoyed anything. Work has become almost unbearable. My job is so futile and monotonous. Sometimes I don't know why they continue to pay me.

February 28
I have this recurring sense that I'm letting everyone down – the people at work, Beth, the kids. We've been spending more money than ever lately, so I have to go on earning it, but I feel guilty every time I see my paycheck.

April 18
This morning I looked in the mirror and I was surprised to see how thin I've gotten. Beth has been nagging me about how little I eat but food just doesn't interest me. I guess I have felt like this a few times before but it seemed as though there was an end in sight. This time I don't understand what the matter is and I don't see any way out.

June 29
I have just realized that nothing interests me and nothing makes me snap out of it. Uncle Charlie's bequest turned out to be $50,000. But what use is money? Beth and I had a fight because she wants to move to a bigger house and I don't see the point.

July 21
Yesterday I took an hour off work and went to Dr. Schwartz. I said I wasn't sleeping. I don't think I got across what was really troubling me. He just said I should go on a vacation and play more golf. I already tried a vacation but it wasn't any fun.

August 4
The mornings are awful. I've been waking up around 5 AM and just lying there. After I'm up I have to force myself to shower and shave. Yesterday I just couldn't do it and I was more than an hour late for work.

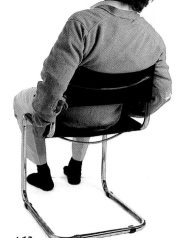

August 13
I don't know what's going to happen to me. Last week I told Mike that I was wasting his time and money working for him. The next day I just didn't get out of bed. In fact, I stayed in bed for 3 days, just thinking how useless I am. Beth called Dr. Schwartz and he sent a psychiatrist over to the house. This guy talked to me for a long time. In the end, he told me that I was depressed. I've known that for a year. He said that I will recover, prescribed some antidepressants, and asked me to come see him in 3 days.

August 27
I started taking the antidepressants but so far they don't seem to help. Dr. Bennett (the psychiatrist) had said they would take a while to work. I've been seeing Dr. Bennett several times a week. We've been talking about some of the changes at work over the past couple of years. He seems to understand what I'm talking about. I feel much better when I talk to him because he listens to me and I'm always surprised how he can explain the things that are happening to me.

October 8
Yesterday on the bus I was thinking about that networking problem at the office and I got so absorbed I missed my stop! I am going back to work next week so I'll have a chance to try out some ideas. I'm seeing Dr. Bennett again today. I know he and I have a long way to go toward working out my problems but I have a sense of progress now. Once the drugs took effect they made a big difference. But I still want to see Dr. Bennett because I think I can get a handle on things now.

MONITOR YOUR SYMPTOMS
ADOLESCENT BEHAVIOR PROBLEMS

Many teenagers challenge the authority symbols and figures in their lives, including parents, schools, and the law. Hormonal changes during puberty cause this behavior in many adolescents as they come to terms with new and disconcerting emotions while making the transition from childhood to adulthood. As the adolescent yearns to be more independent, arguments with parents are typical and are generally not a cause for serious concern. Healthy family relationships usually survive the turbulent adolescent years without permanent damage. Occasionally, though, an adolescent displays serious behavior problems that require professional supervision.

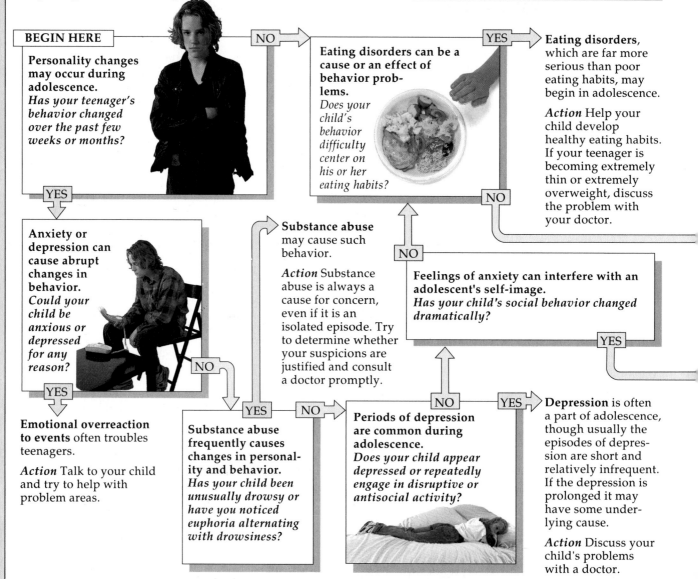

WARNING

The following signs may indicate that your child has been abusing drugs:

◆ Slurred and confused speech
◆ Lack of coordination and balance
◆ Drowsiness and lethargy alternating with euphoria or hyperactivity
◆ Excessive eating or shivering
◆ Heavy or "droopy" eyelids
◆ Abnormally large or small pupils
◆ Loss of weight and/or appetite
◆ Violent mood swings
◆ Alcohol on the breath

BEGIN HERE
NO →
YES →

Personality changes may occur during adolescence.
Has your teenager's behavior changed over the past few weeks or months?

Eating disorders can be a cause or an effect of behavior problems.
Does your child's behavior difficulty center on his or her eating habits?

Eating disorders, which are far more serious than poor eating habits, may begin in adolescence.

Action Help your child develop healthy eating habits. If your teenager is becoming extremely thin or extremely overweight, discuss the problem with your doctor.

YES ↓
NO

Anxiety or depression can cause abrupt changes in behavior.
Could your child be anxious or depressed for any reason?

Substance abuse may cause such behavior.

Action Substance abuse is always a cause for concern, even if it is an isolated episode. Try to determine whether your suspicions are justified and consult a doctor promptly.

NO

Feelings of anxiety can interfere with an adolescent's self-image.
Has your child's social behavior changed dramatically?

YES

YES ↓
NO

Emotional overreaction to events often troubles teenagers.

Action Talk to your child and try to help with problem areas.

YES   NO →

Substance abuse frequently causes changes in personality and behavior.
Has your child been unusually drowsy or have you noticed euphoria alternating with drowsiness?

Periods of depression are common during adolescence.
Does your child appear depressed or repeatedly engage in disruptive or antisocial activity?

NO   YES →

Depression is often a part of adolescence, though usually the episodes of depression are short and relatively infrequent. If the depression is prolonged it may have some underlying cause.

Action Discuss your child's problems with a doctor.

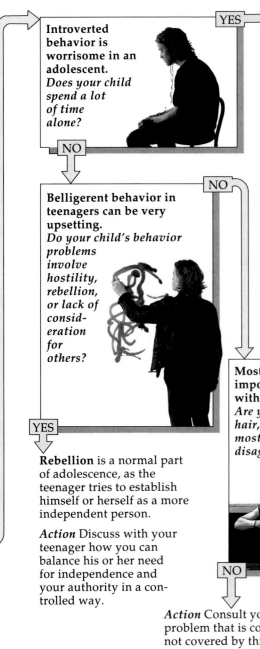

Introverted behavior is worrisome in an adolescent.
Does your child spend a lot of time alone?

NO

YES

Shyness is common in adolescence as the teenager struggles with his or her social identity and adulthood. Occasionally, however, a child feels isolated because of deeper anxiety or fear.

Action Talk to your child about his or her shyness and try to provide plenty of nonthreatening opportunities to socialize. If you identify a problem, such as self-consciousness about being overweight or having acne, try to help.

Belligerent behavior in teenagers can be very upsetting.
Do your child's behavior problems involve hostility, rebellion, or lack of consideration for others?

NO

YES

Rebellion is a normal part of adolescence, as the teenager tries to establish himself or herself as a more independent person.

Action Discuss with your teenager how you can balance his or her need for independence and your authority in a controlled way.

Most teenagers find it important to identify with their peer group.
Are your child's clothes, hair, and/or language the most frequent cause of disagreement?

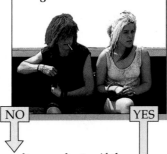

NO

YES

Action Consult your doctor if the problem that is concerning you is not covered by this chart.

Anxiety may take many forms, ranging from aggression and rudeness to over-dependence.

Action Talk to your child to try to identify and understand the source of the anxiety. If you can establish the cause, try to reassure your child and discuss ways of resolving the problem.

Peer-group identification gives the teenager a sense of belonging to a group; growing away from the family, the teenager wants to identify with another group for security. Extreme styles of language, dress, or behavior can be disconcerting but are not generally a cause for concern unless they are associated with substance abuse or other illegal activities.

Action Ignore your child's behavior as much as possible, unless it is causing trouble at school or at home. Most adolescents tone down their dress and behavior as they grow older.

ASK YOUR DOCTOR
SIGNS OF MENTAL PROBLEMS

Q My daughter has lost so much weight that her clothes do not fit her. She still says she is too fat and insists on buying larger sizes than she needs. Should I let her keep dieting?

A Talk to your doctor or a psychiatrist immediately. Serious eating disorders such as anorexia nervosa or bulimia (the binge-purge syndrome) develop in 5 to 12 percent of adolescents. Your daughter's unrealistic concern about her weight may indicate serious emotional conflict.

Q My son checks to make sure his bedroom windows are closed at least 20 times a day. Does he have some mental problem?

A Discuss the situation with your doctor, who may recommend psychiatric evaluation. A psychoanalyst would recommend therapy for emotional problems that express themselves as obsessive-compulsive behavior. A behavior therapist would try to modify your son's actions without probing into emotional causes.

Q When my husband is "up," he is a big spender, lavishing me with gifts. But often by the time the bill comes, he is berating himself for putting us in a bad financial spot. Why does he do this?

A Your husband's behavior may indicate bipolar depression, characterized by disruptive mood swings. A person with this disorder may alternate between periods of elation and deep depression. Talk to your doctor or a psychiatrist; treatment may involve antidepressant medication and psychiatric help.

PANIC DISORDER AND SUICIDE

About 1.5 percent of the US population have experienced a panic disorder (persistent, repeated panic attacks) at some time in their lives; occasional panic attacks affect two to three times more people. A recent study unexpectedly showed that people with panic disorders attempted suicide at an even higher rate than people with major depressions. This greater incidence of suicide attempts was independent of other factors such as alcohol or other drug abuse or depression.

SUICIDE AND ATTEMPTED SUICIDE

Suicide or suicide attempts are among the most tragic reactions to emotional disorders. Most people who commit suicide suffer from depression or anxiety disorders, or abuse alcohol or other drugs. A very few "impulsive" suicides occur after some catastrophic event.

What are the usual reasons?

The reasons for suicide are many and complex. The most common is the desire to escape from personal despair when the individual cannot see any relief other than death. However, some people appear to commit suicide out of anger, to make others feel guilty, or because they genuinely believe people would be better off without them. Others feel guilty and deserving of punishment. It is not always possible to explain a person's motives satisfactorily after suicide.

Major depression is the leading cause of suicide. The symptoms of depression may disrupt relationships or result in failures in school or work. Personal problems may precede a suicide attempt, but they are consequences of depression rather than causes of suicide.

How common is suicide?

The incidence of suicide varies widely throughout the world. The published figures may not always present a true picture because suicide is sometimes difficult to distinguish from accidental death or is intentionally misreported.

In the US, more than 30,000 people commit suicide each year and about 250,000 attempt to do so. Another 250,000 people communicate an intention to commit suicide without actually doing it. In all countries, suicide rates are higher among men than women. Men succeed in killing themselves three times as often as women. However, a suicide attempt carried out in a manner unlikely to succeed, sometimes as a plea for help, is more common in women. More than 75 percent of those who commit suicide in the US are male; 60 to 70 percent of those who attempt suicide are female. A partial explanation may be that men have difficulty expressing their feelings, leading to a built-up inner turmoil. Women have a "safety valve" because in many cases they more readily express their feelings. The rate of attempted suicide seems to peak between the ages of 15 and 30. People over 40 have a higher rate of actual suicide. Older people may commit suicide as a result of accumulated disappointments and despair.

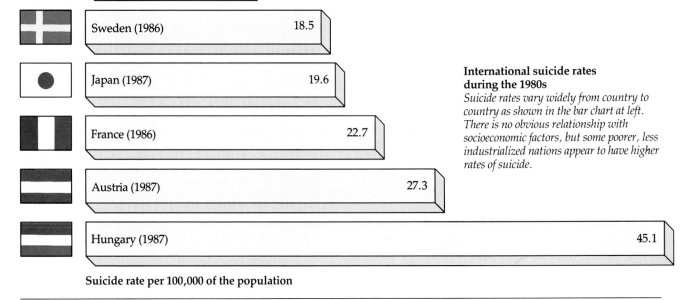

UK (1987) 8.1
US (1987) 12.7
Sweden (1986) 18.5
Japan (1987) 19.6
France (1986) 22.7
Austria (1987) 27.3
Hungary (1987) 45.1

Suicide rate per 100,000 of the population

International suicide rates during the 1980s
Suicide rates vary widely from country to country as shown in the bar chart at left. There is no obvious relationship with socioeconomic factors, but some poorer, less industrialized nations appear to have higher rates of suicide.

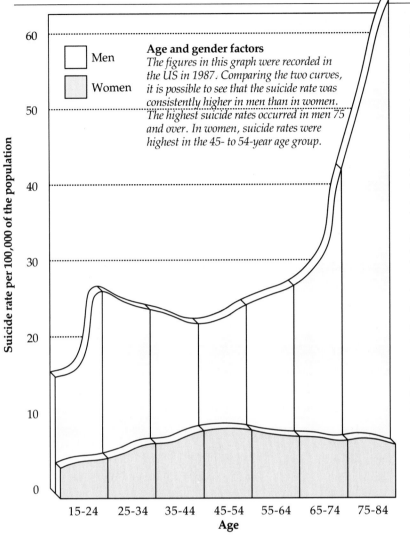

Age and gender factors
The figures in this graph were recorded in the US in 1987. Comparing the two curves, it is possible to see that the suicide rate was consistently higher in men than in women. The highest suicide rates occurred in men 75 and over. In women, suicide rates were highest in the 45- to 54-year age group.

Suicide among adolescents has increased over the last 30 years. A 1987 study showed that 14 percent of eighth to tenth graders attempt suicide and 34 percent say they have seriously thought about it. Like adults, suicidal adolescents are often depressed. The same study reported that 61 percent of adolescents feel sad and hopeless. The reasons for the increasing suicide rate among young people are still not known.

Can suicide be prevented?

No one can surely predict suicide, but there are a number of risk factors and warning signs that you can be aware of (see box below). Any threat of suicide should be taken seriously. If someone is talking to you about a desire to commit suicide, follow these guidelines:

◆ Never lecture or attempt to advise the person. Listen attentively and provide reassurance that effective treatment for depression is available.

◆ Consult a psychiatrist immediately so that the person can receive treatment.

◆ Remove any objects that could be used to commit suicide.

RISK FACTORS AND WARNING SIGNS

The following factors and warning signs may alert you that someone you know is at risk of suicide.

◆ **A history of previous attempts.** In a person whose self-esteem is already low, failure to succeed at suicide may be taken as even further evidence of worthlessness.

◆ **A suicide by a close friend or family member.** Young people often copy the behavior of those closest to them.

◆ **A serious or overwhelming medical problem.** Incurable cancer or AIDS, for example, can lead to suicide.

◆ **A history of threats or a sudden threat of suicide.** The person may express the wish to be dead and describe methods of achieving this end.

◆ **Prolonged or recurrent episodes of depression.** Prolonged depression is especially likely to lead to suicide when it is associated with physical symptoms, increasing social withdrawal, and rejection of help.

◆ **Alcohol or other drug abuse.** Many attempted suicides occur after drinking alcohol.

◆ **A sudden, inexplicable lightening of mood after a period of depression.** This can sometimes signal a person's final resolve to commit suicide.

◆ **Availability of the means.** Access to guns or drugs increases the risk of suicide in a depressed person.

◆ **Loss of a partner.** Divorced and widowed people are more at risk than either single or married people.

◆ **The withdrawal of social support.** Discharge from medical treatment, for example, may trigger suicide.

◆ **Perception of deprivation.** Setbacks such as losing a job can precipitate suicide. Times of celebration are peak risk times because the suicidal person contrasts his or her unhappiness with the supposed happiness of others and feels emotionally deprived.

CHAPTER FOUR

MONITOR YOUR LIFE-STYLE

IN EARLIER TIMES, people may have had good reason to feel fatalistic about illness, believing that sickness struck at random. Advances in health care have altered that point of view forever. Today an individual has a much larger measure of control over his or her health. Now that medical science has eliminated or controlled almost all of the bacterial infections (such as typhoid, tuberculosis, meningitis, and pneumonia) that decimated earlier generations, how long you can expect to live and how healthy you remain has become more a matter of choice and less one of chance. Many of the crippling or fatal disorders of the late 20th century are caused or accelerated by our living habits. Factors such as inherited genetic predispositions are also relevant, but these (unlike some environmental factors and our habits) cannot

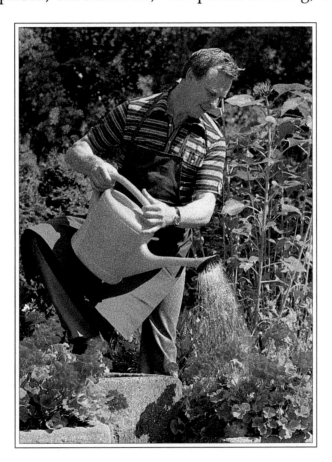

be changed. Everyone can minimize his or her risk of illness by following a health-promoting way of life. In this chapter, we describe the influences of a whole range of factors, beginning with the important issue of psychological stress. We explain the difference between healthy stress (which motivates us and spurs us into action) and unhealthy stress (which interferes with our functioning efficiently and may damage our health). We tell you how you can learn to recognize the warning signs of unhealthy, unproductive stress.

The type of work you do can affect both your emotional and physical health. We draw your attention to the risks to which you might be exposed in the office, in some industries, or in jobs involving animals. We tell you when protection, such as special clothing, is essential and which jobs may require you to have regular tests to detect early signs of disease. We then look at the impact on health of where we live and the risks that may be associated with traveling to or living in an environment to which we are not adapted. We also examine the important area of sexuality. Our attitudes toward sex can influence our emotional happiness and our sexual behavior can seriously affect our physical health. Finally, we look at alcohol and tobacco – the two main causes of premature death in the US. Alcohol is linked with one in every 20 deaths, including deaths from medical conditions, traffic accidents, homicides, suicides, and (nontraffic) accidents. Tobacco is linked with one third of all cancers and is a major cause of coronary heart disease. Knowledge of the effects of these habits can help guide you to a healthier life.

YOUR STRESS LEVEL

A SIMPLE DEFINITION of stress is an event or circumstance that requires you to adapt. We all require a certain amount of stress to stimulate and motivate us in our work and recreational or social activities. However, stress can become damaging when demands become greater than you can cope with.

Stress can have both short-term and long-term effects, which can be either helpful or harmful. The immediate effects of stress on the body (an overall arousal response) are beneficial in their original context – that is, to prepare the body for effective action. This "fight or flight" response (see illustration) is caused by the effects of the sympathetic nervous system on many parts of the body and by the release of stress hormones into the bloodstream. Such a response is appropriate for physical exertion (for example, when a sprinter is anticipating the start of a race). However, when the physical effects of stress occur repeatedly and in situations where they have no useful effect (such as in response to frustration or psychological pressures), a person's physical and mental health can be adversely affected. Some people are more susceptible than others to stress-related medical problems.

THE "FIGHT OR FLIGHT" RESPONSE

The hypothalamus sets a number of events in motion that are described below. Your body responds immediately (see illustration).

Chemical signals that are carried in the bloodstream stimulate part of the adrenal gland (the cortex) to release cortisol, a hormone. Cortisol circulates through your body via the bloodstream; it is particularly important in immune system function.

Nerve signals are sent down the spinal cord to increase the activity of the sympathetic nerves. These nerves are part of the autonomic (involuntary) nervous system, which regulates many body functions, including breathing.

Nerve signals stimulate another part of the adrenal gland (the medulla) to release the hormones epinephrine and norepinephrine. Epinephrine increases the speed and force of the heartbeat; norepinephrine maintains blood pressure.

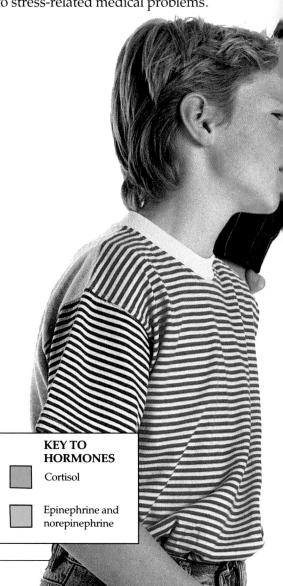

KEY TO HORMONES

Cortisol

Epinephrine and norepinephrine

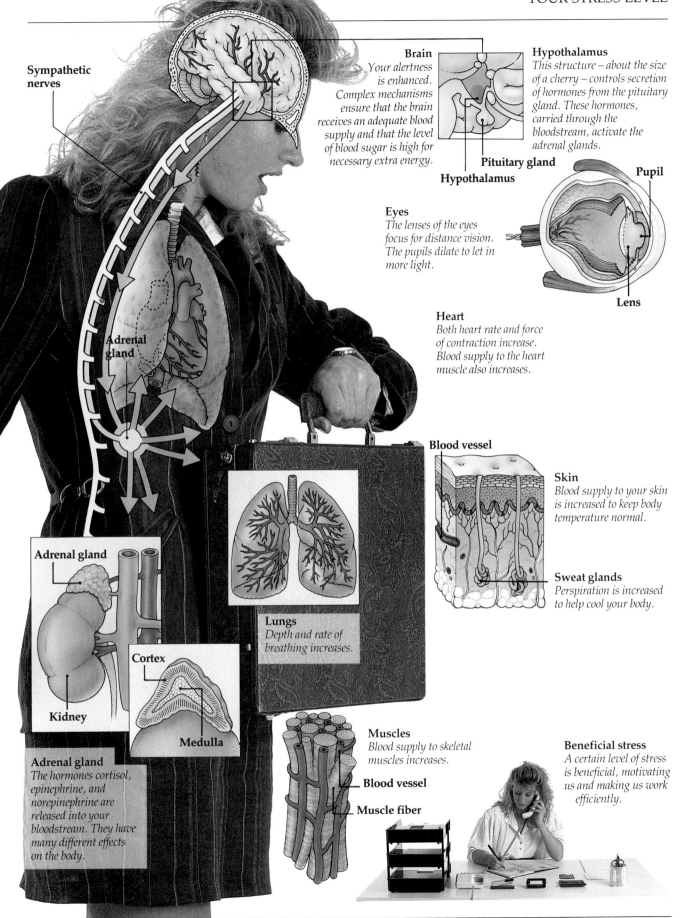

Sympathetic nerves

Brain
Your alertness is enhanced. Complex mechanisms ensure that the brain receives an adequate blood supply and that the level of blood sugar is high for necessary extra energy.

Hypothalamus
This structure – about the size of a cherry – controls secretion of hormones from the pituitary gland. These hormones, carried through the bloodstream, activate the adrenal glands.

Pituitary gland

Hypothalamus

Pupil

Eyes
The lenses of the eyes focus for distance vision. The pupils dilate to let in more light.

Lens

Heart
Both heart rate and force of contraction increase. Blood supply to the heart muscle also increases.

Adrenal gland

Blood vessel

Skin
Blood supply to your skin is increased to keep body temperature normal.

Sweat glands
Perspiration is increased to help cool your body.

Adrenal gland

Kidney

Cortex

Medulla

Lungs
Depth and rate of breathing increases.

Adrenal gland
The hormones cortisol, epinephrine, and norepinephrine are released into your bloodstream. They have many different effects on the body.

Muscles
Blood supply to skeletal muscles increases.

Blood vessel

Muscle fiber

Beneficial stress
A certain level of stress is beneficial, motivating us and making us work efficiently.

89

WHEN CAN STRESS BE DAMAGING?

Whether stress is damaging or not depends mainly on the level of demands imposed, the person's ability to cope, and any physical effects. Evidence suggests that negative stress (such as a natural disaster or an argument) rather than positive, enjoyable stimulation (such as getting married or winning a prize) has a detrimental effect on your health.

Individual perception is also important. An event that is highly threatening to one person may be entirely manageable or even enjoyable to someone else. This difference in perception may result partly from life experiences and partly from attitude.

Situations that cause stress are more likely to be damaging if you cannot predict or control them. This factor is particularly apparent where job stress is concerned. Highly demanding jobs are much more stressful if the individual has no control over the workload, as on a factory assembly line on which the work is paced by the speed of the line. Conversely, an executive's job may not be harmfully stressful if he or she has the freedom to plan and control the work.

Stress is more likely to have adverse effects if you lack social support (if you have no one in whom you can confide) or if you have personal, financial, or other immediate concerns.

Prolonged, repeated, or major stress

If you are subjected to several sources of major stress (see the SCALE OF LIFE EVENTS on page 91) or severely prolonged minor stress (such as daily frustrations), your body experiences repeated or prolonged physical changes. Although you may not be aware of any physical effects, your body may be experiencing a constant state of agitation. Different organs and systems throughout your body can be

---

WARNING

If you experience any of the following symptoms you could be under stress:

- Breathlessness
- Palpitations
- Nausea or vomiting
- Dizziness
- Loss of appetite
- Constant hunger
- Insomnia
- Nightmares
- Constant tiredness or fatigue
- Onset of allergies
- Chronic indigestion
- Constipation or diarrhea
- Headaches
- Neck or backaches
- Impotence
- Clumsiness
- Trembling
- Hot flashes

HEALTHY STRESS

Effective
Creative
Constructive

Joyful
Exuberant
Curious

High

Performance level

UNHEALTHY STRESS

Bored
Lacking motivation

Tense
Overcompetitive
Fearful
Depressed

Low

Low   Stress level   High

Healthy and unhealthy stress
A certain amount of stress enables you to live a stimulating and enjoyable life. However, too much stress, as indicated on the right side of the graph, has a harmful effect on your mind and body.

affected. The immune system may be weakened, thus reducing the body's ability to resist infection. Many people visit doctors with physical complaints that are related to stress. Long-term stress can also lead to serious psychological and psychiatric problems, such as panic attacks (see page 80) and other anxiety disorders. In extreme cases, long-term stress can lead to a so-called nervous breakdown, in which the person is unable to function on a day-to-day basis because of emotional problems.

Signs and symptoms of stress

You may experience any of a number of physical symptoms of stress (see WARNING on page 90), many of which are similar to those of anxiety disorders and/or depression. You may suffer mental, emotional, or personality deterioration (see SIGNS OF MENTAL PROBLEMS on page 78). The way you function – at work or at home – may deteriorate. You may become a heavy user of alcohol or other drugs, including cigarettes, in an attempt to reduce the effects of stress.

EFFECTS OF STRESS

Stress may contribute to the occurrence of:

♦ Anxiety disorders, phobias, or other mental illnesses
♦ Asthma
♦ Migraines
♦ Ulcers
♦ Hypertension
♦ Stroke
♦ Heart disease
♦ Cancer

SCALE OF LIFE EVENTS

Much of the research on major, prolonged, or repeated stress comes from studying people's responses to stressful situations. One well-known scale of life events – the Social Readjustment Rating Scale – evaluates the effects of events that require an individual to adapt. Use the table below (showing selected items from the scale) to determine your score in "life-change units." Check every item that you have experienced in the last 18 months. Then add up the life-change units. If your total score is more than 200, you are likely to be experiencing significant physical or mental effects of stress.

LIFE EVENT	Life-change units
Death of spouse or partner	100
Divorce	73
Marital separation	65
Death of a close family member	63
Personal injury or illness	53
Marriage	50
Being fired	47
Retirement	45
Change in health of family member	44
Pregnancy	40
Sex problems; addition of family member; business readjustment	39
Dramatic change in financial status	38
Death of a close friend	37
Change to different type of work	36
Foreclosure of mortgage or loan	30
Outstanding personal achievement	28
Beginning or ending school; spouse or partner begins or stops work	26
Trouble with boss	23
Change in work hours or conditions; change in residence or schools	20
Change in social activities	18
Change in sleeping habits	16
Vacation	13
Major holiday	12
Minor violations of the law	11

MANAGING STRESS BY MANAGING TIME

The ability to use time effectively is one way to help manage stress. If you often feel tense and anxious because you fall behind with everyday tasks, you may be able to improve your time-management skills. Try the approaches suggested below:

Identify your problems

Prepare a daily action list over the course of a week to see how you are coping with your work load. Write down any problems that interfered with your tasks or prevented you from completing them. Once you have identified your time-management problems, you will be in a better position to control them.

Improve your time-planning technique

One of the most effective ways to address your daily stresses is to thoroughly plan the time you have. Spend at least 15 minutes each day organizing your work and assigning priorities in a daily planner such as the one shown at right. Use symbols to indicate the priority of each task and the stage of completion you have reached. Transfer all uncompleted work to the next day's list and record any more insights you have. Remember that challenges may arise that require your immediate attention, temporarily superseding other responsibilities.

Avoid procrastination

Procrastination is a time-wasting habit. Try the following tips to make yourself more productive. Turn unwelcome tasks into challenges and offer yourself rewards. Decide on the best time of day for the type of work required. Tackle the most difficult job first. Split overwhelming projects into more manageable chunks.

DAILY PLANNER Date: *July 5th*

Time	APPOINTMENTS AND SCHEDULED EVENTS	Place
AM 11:30	Meeting to discuss new project with Susan.	Conference Room.
PM 1:00	Lunch with Bob Moore, data resources.	Meet at his office.

TO BE DONE TODAY   (Prioritized daily action list)

1. Read reports from last week's meeting. I →
2. Prepare agenda for Monday.   ✳ ✓
3. Prepare presentation graphics + letter. ✳ ✓
4. Review job applications and schedule interviews.   I ✓
5. Pick up clothes from dry cleaners.   →
6. Buy red wine for dinner tonight.   ✳ ✓

1. Too many telephone interruptions – ask Andy D to help out or have calls held for at least an hour.
2. Too much paperwork – must organize my ✳ working files.

KEY	✳ urgent D delegated → carried over
	I important ✓ completed

EIGHT WAYS TO CONTROL STRESS

 Talk about your problems. When tension builds, discuss your problems with a close friend, your partner, or the people at the source of a problem.

 Learn to relax completely. Take time every day to rest – even if only for a few minutes. Close your eyes, relax your body, and clear your mind of concerns.

 Exercise regularly. Try different types of exercise and develop a consistent exercise routine that you can really enjoy and maintain.

 Take regular breaks. Take a short break to refresh your mind after a period of concentrated effort or when you are frustrated with a project.

 Avoid too many changes at once. Whenever possible, plan for the future to ensure that major life changes do not occur simultaneously.

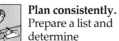 **Plan consistently.** Prepare a list and determine priorities each day to gain control of your work load and prevent frustration.

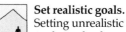 **Set realistic goals.** Setting unrealistic goals can lead to frustration. Be practical about what you can accomplish.

 See your doctor if necessary. If the stress in your life becomes intolerable, do not hesitate to talk to your doctor about your concerns.

CASE HISTORY
A STRESSFUL LIFE-STYLE

KAREN IS A BUSY **audiologist for a public school system. She was recently promoted to the managerial position she always wanted. But soon Karen became troubled by fatigue and loss of energy. At home, her family noticed that she was more irritable than usual, and that she was often too tired to enjoy family activities. Her husband Don suggested that she see her doctor about her fatigue and listlessness.**

PERSONAL DETAILS
Name Karen Bennett
Age 36
Occupation Audiologist
Family Married; two children, 10 and 12.

THE CONSULTATION

Karen's family doctor questions her and learns that, in addition to fatigue, Karen has been having abdominal discomfort, especially after meals. Karen also tells the doctor that she has little interest in sex.

The doctor takes a detailed medical history, carries out a complete physical examination, and arranges for Karen to have blood tests and a gynecological checkup. However, all the test results are negative, and there appears to be no indication of any physical disorder.

FURTHER INVESTIGATION

The doctor questions Karen in more detail about her life-style. She discovers that Karen's daily routine is extremely demanding. On her way to work she has to go out of her way to take the children to school and then must drive through heavy, congested traffic. At work, she often feels the need to stay late to review new procedures, but doing so interferes with picking up the children.

She also wants to get home in time to prepare the evening meal for her family. By the time she prepares dinner and cleans up, the evening is almost over. Although Karen was once a regular swimmer and tennis player, she has not exercised in months and can't find time for other leisure activities or interests.

THE DIAGNOSIS

Until she talked to her doctor, Karen had not realized how complicated her life had become. She is not surprised when her doctor says her symptoms are probably caused by STRESS. The doctor says that Karen's promotion may have helped strain her already overloaded schedule to the breaking point.

THE TREATMENT

Karen's doctor helps her set her priorities and determine some realistic plans for allocating her time. Through her children's school, Karen joins a working parents' support group, and she and other group members talk over solutions to some of the everyday problems that they encounter. Karen also sets aside two nights and one morning a week for exercise classes, which she attends with one of her friends. Don and the children agree to make their own meals at those times.

THE FOLLOW-UP

As she adjusts to her new responsibilities at work, Karen's anxiety subsides and she has more energy to enjoy her family life and her activities with friends. She begins to feel the benefits of exercise and the relief from her daily schedule as family cook and chauffeur. She and a woman from the support group now share the services of a high school student who picks up their children from school and watches them twice a week. Karen's mental and physical health are better than ever.

Reducing stress through exercise
Karen finds that attending an exercise class several times a week helps relieve tension.

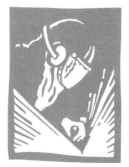

YOUR JOB

GREAT STRIDES have been made in the past 75 years in the areas of occupational safety and health. In the US, work-related deaths have been reduced 80 percent in that time, even though the work force has expanded steadily. The risks of some occupations, such as construction work or mining, are obvious or implied and must be assumed as a condition of employment. But the hazards are far better understood and managed today than in the past.

SMOKING AND OCCUPATIONAL DISEASES

Tobacco smoke is itself a carcinogen. It can also enhance the carcinogenic qualities of other substances to increase the risk of lung cancer. Evidence is particularly strong of such an effect between asbestos and smoking.

The introduction of national safety and health regulations, sophisticated monitoring systems, and regular medical surveillance of employees has substantially reduced the risk of occupational disease and injury. In the US, the incidence of occupational disease is relatively low compared to many other countries. Even so, significant numbers of workers, particularly in construction and manufacturing jobs, are diagnosed as having work-related diseases. Work accidents, including many motor-vehicle accidents and falls, injure workers as well.

OCCUPATIONAL DISEASES

Occupational diseases may result from exposure to chemical, organic, or physical agents or from other contributing factors in the workplace.

Dust inhalation

Prolonged inhalation of mineral dusts may lead to fibrosis of the lungs, which causes the lungs to stiffen and lose their elasticity. The most prevalent form of fibrosis is asbestosis, caused by the in-

Protecting against dust inhalation
Engineering controls (e.g., adequate ventilation and the use of masks approved by the National Institute for Occupational Safety and Health) offer respiratory protection to workers exposed to dust. The mask shown here is used to protect against asbestos fibers and other harmful substances. Asbestos workers must also wear protective clothing and the work area must be sealed off from other workers and the general public.

Testing for lung damage
Workers exposed to potentially harmful dusts should have regular chest X-rays to detect early signs of respiratory disease. This color-enhanced X-ray shows early signs of silicosis, a lung disease caused by inhaling dust containing silica. Tests of an individual's lung function may also be performed. Because dust diseases develop over a period of many years, workers should have regular tests and X-rays throughout their lives.

halation of asbestos fibers. Asbestosis is currently one of the most common occupational diseases diagnosed in the US. Exposure to asbestos is also a factor in the development of lung cancer. Other common forms of fibrosis are caused by inhaling coal dust or dust containing silica. Exposure to a number of synthetic chemicals used in the manufacture of paints and plastics may also induce fibrosis. Inhalation of organic dusts that contain fungal spores can lead to farmers' lung, a type of pneumonia.

Chemical-related diseases

Many industrial chemicals can damage the respiratory system, including the lungs, if inhaled. If they are absorbed into the bloodstream through the lungs or skin or if they are ingested, they may damage other organs. Contact with the skin may irritate or destroy the skin or cause an allergic response. Many chemicals are associated with an increased risk of lung, bladder, bone marrow, and skin cancer. Workers who are exposed to chemicals should have regular blood, liver function, and/or urine tests.

Radiation-linked diseases

Ionizing radiation includes alpha particles, which can be stopped by skin but are harmful if inhaled; beta rays, which can penetrate the skin and alter internal tissues; and gamma rays, which are similar to X-rays and can be stopped by dense materials such as lead. Exposure to ionizing radiation can affect people in the nuclear power and nuclear weapons industries, and in medicine

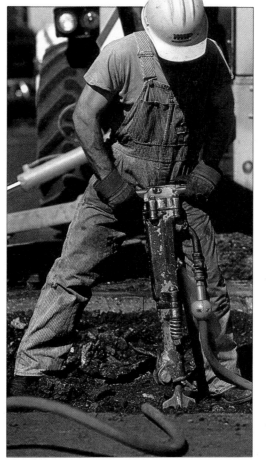

Noise damage
Hearing loss caused by prolonged exposure to loud noise is one of the most common occupational disorders, after lung diseases. Wearing earmuffs or earplugs and limiting the length of exposure to the noise may reduce the risk of damage. Workers at risk should have regular hearing tests.

Vibration damage
Exposure to vibration from the use of hand-held tools may lead to Raynaud's phenomenon, in which the neuromuscular regulation of the vessels in the hands and fingers is altered. Another prevalent disorder is carpal tunnel syndrome, in which the nerves to the palm and fingers are injured where they pass through a channel in the wrist.

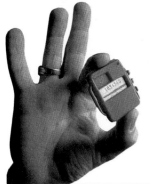

Radiation monitor
People at risk of exposure to ionizing radiation are required to wear special badges that monitor cumulative exposure. One such device consists of a piece of photographic film inside a holder. The film, which darkens in response to radiation, is checked periodically.

WORK INJURIES

The National Institute for Occupational Safety and Health estimates that at least 10 million people experience job-related injuries each year; 3 million of the injuries are considered severe. Many injuries are permanently disabling. Most workplaces have clear-cut safety regulations and controls. A safety program that significantly reduces on-the-job injuries requires the cooperation of both management and employees. Your positive attitude toward safety may prevent injury to yourself or a coworker. In addition, you can reduce the possibility of an accident by following these guidelines:

◆ Always follow safety procedures.
◆ Wear protective clothing, if required. For example, construction workers should always wear hard hats on the work site.
◆ If you are taking any prescribed or over-the-counter medication, check with your doctor about potential side effects, such as drowsiness, that could make it dangerous for you to perform your work activities.
◆ If your job requires you to operate potentially dangerous machinery, be sure that you are well-rested and alert on the job.

and research, as well as people undergoing diagnostic or therapeutic procedures. Exposure to sunlight is the most widespread source of nonionizing radiation. This type of radiation can penetrate only superficial layers of body tissue.

Infectious diseases

People who work with animals – including workers in food manufacturing and farming – may be at risk of contracting an infectious disease. For example, psittacosis, a form of pneumonia, may be acquired from birds. If birds and livestock are checked regularly by a veterinarian, such diseases can be prevented. Leptospirosis, which often causes kidney and liver damage, is transmitted in the urine of infected rats; farmers and sewer workers may be at risk. Any worker in whom symptoms develop should promptly seek a doctor's advice.

OFFICE HEALTH HAZARDS

Though occupational health risks for the office worker remain comparatively low, a number of significant health considerations have recently come to light. Many of these are associated with structural features of the modern office building (such as lighting, heating, or ventilation systems) or with the use of office equipment such as copiers and video display terminals (VDTs).

Muscle fatigue, backache, eye fatigue, and repetitive motion injury to arms or hands caused by prolonged keyboard work are common complaints among VDT operators. The relative heights of your chair, desk, and keyboard may contribute to fatigue. Looking at the screen poses no apparent risk of injury to your eyes or vision, but have any existing eye problems checked.

RISKS TO HEALTH CARE WORKERS

Health care workers are at risk of hepatitis B and AIDS as a result of exposure to blood or other body fluids. There are special procedures for the safe handling of blood, needles, and blood products. Vaccination helps protect against hepatitis B.

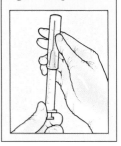

SICK BUILDING SYNDROME

Sick building syndrome refers to a group of symptoms sometimes experienced by people who live or work in modern homes or office buildings served by closed ventilation systems. It is a phenomenon recently recognized by the United Nations and the National Institute for Occupational Safety and Health. The exact cause of the syndrome has, in many instances, not been identified. A combination of environmental factors, including recycled tobacco smoke, microorganisms, climate, and airborne levels of carbon monoxide, probably causes the problem. Identifying and clearing up the sources of indoor pollutants, adequately cleaning and regulating ventilation systems, and regulating temperature seem to reduce the symptoms in many instances. Some people who have symptoms may benefit from medication; for others, a job change is the only solution. Treatment usually focuses on correcting the problem with the building rather than on medical care for the individual.

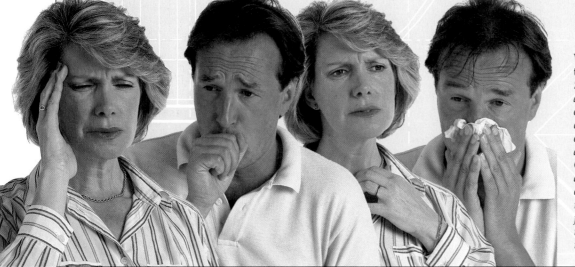

What are the symptoms?
Sick building syndrome affects people in a variety of ways. The most common complaint is of extreme tiredness, often accompanied by headache. Other symptoms include a blocked or runny nose, eye irritation, rashes, nausea, and mental fatigue. Asthma develops in some people working in certain buildings.

HOW TO REDUCE THE HAZARDS IN YOUR OFFICE

Rest your eyes
Eye fatigue can result from prolonged focus on a VDT screen, as well as glare from extraneous light sources. A periodic break every 20 to 30 minutes during which you intentionally focus on distant objects will help alleviate the strain on your eye muscles. Filters are available to help reduce the glare on the screen.

Avoid repetitive motion
If aches develop in your hands and/or arms, switch to another task until the symptoms have subsided. If you experience pain, talk to your doctor. If necessary, ask to be transferred to another job that does not involve similar types of motion. The discomfort caused by repetitive motion can be alleviated only by resting the affected part of the body.

Adjust lighting
Flickering fluorescent lighting causes anxiety and headaches in some people. Background lighting is not always adequate. An adjustable desk lamp may help.

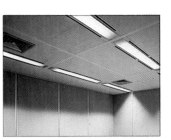

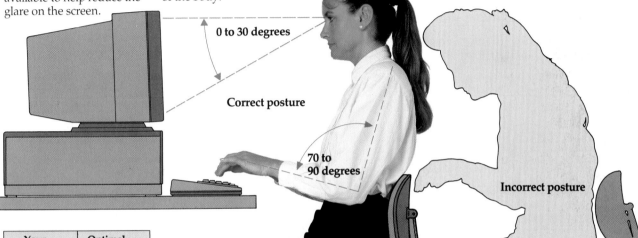

0 to 30 degrees

Correct posture

70 to 90 degrees

Incorrect posture

Your height	Optimal desk height
4'11"	23"
5'4"	24"
5'6"	25"
5'9"	26"
6'2"	28"

Adjust desk height
The height of your desk should enable you to sit at a keyboard so that your lower arms form a 70- to 90-degree angle to your torso. The monitor should be within a 30-degree viewing angle of your direct line of vision. Use the table above to check your desk height.

Avoid tobacco smoke
Tobacco smoke is harmful not only to the smoker but to his or her coworkers. There is now evidence that tobacco smoke increases the risk of lung cancer among coworkers. Tobacco smoke may also contribute to sick building syndrome. Many offices and hospitals have established a smoke-free working environment to protect the work force from smoke hazards.

Regulate temperature
In a large office, you may not be able to control heating or air conditioning, although you may ask for adjustments. Your comfort depends on a combination of factors, including temperature, humidity, air velocity, clothing, and the task you are performing. You may be able to adjust one or more of these factors.

Adjust seating
Poor posture is one of the factors that contribute to backache and eye fatigue. Adjust your chair to suit your height at the desk and to provide sufficient support for your lower back. The height of your chair should enable you to sit in a relaxed position with your feet firmly on the floor and your back straight. A foot rest may be necessary if your chair is too high and its height cannot be adjusted sufficiently.

YOUR ENVIRONMENT

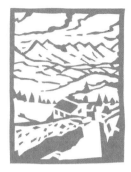

THE ENVIRONMENT in which we live makes a significant impact on our lives. The environment affects our health, our quality of life, and our state of mind. Some of the factors that affect health are naturally occurring phenomena, such as climate and altitude. Others are the result of human activity, such as industrial pollution, auto emissions, and tobacco smoke.

POLLEN COUNTS

Some types of asthma and hay fever are the body's response to pollens in the atmosphere. People with these types of asthma and hay fever should monitor the pollen count and, if necessary, avoid going outdoors on days when the pollen count is particularly high. Air filters help clean indoor air.

Human beings are amazingly adaptable. We are able to live in many types of environments, ranging from the cold steppes of Russia to the rain forests of South America. However, if we go to visit or live in other regions, we may experience severe discomfort or even become seriously ill, especially if we have not prepared for the differences.

THE AIR WE BREATHE

Air is vital. Yet, in many areas of the world, pollution makes the air we breathe damaging to our health. Common illnesses such as bronchitis and asthma can be aggravated by living in polluted areas. Inefficient burning of fossil fuels has been a major factor in the development of chronic bronchitis in industrialized countries. Controls that are now being enforced may eventually improve the situation and result in better air quality.

People with any type of chest disease should definitely avoid situations where they might be exposed to tobacco smoke. If possible, they should live in low-pollution areas where levels of automobile exhaust fumes and industrial pollution are lower.

CONTRIBUTING TO A BETTER ENVIRONMENT

People are increasingly aware of the need to reduce pollution in the environment and to conserve natural resources. You can contribute to a safer, healthier environment by taking the following steps.

Provide your own power
Walking or using a bicycle instead of a car for short trips saves gas, cuts down on pollution, and also helps keep you in shape. Many areas have special bicycle paths.

Recycle
Separate items such as cans, bottles, and newspapers from the rest of your garbage and take them to a recycling center. Your city or town may already have established a recycling program.

Use public transportation
If your area has a good public transportation system, take advantage of it. You will help reduce pollution and traffic congestion.

SOURCES OF ENVIRONMENTAL POLLUTION

Industrial processes, automobile emissions, sewage, aerosols, pesticides, and tobacco smoke are among the sources of pollution that threaten public health in an industrialized nation. Efforts to reduce pollution are costly and complex, requiring fundamental changes in farming, industry, and individual life-style.

Water pollution

Water may be polluted by bacterial contamination – for example, from untreated sewage. Pollution can also occur from the seeping of agricultural chemicals into our water supplies. In developed countries, water quality is generally carefully monitored, and the public is usually warned about contaminants.

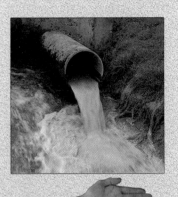

Auto emissions

Carbon monoxide and lead are among the most dangerous pollutants in the emissions that come from automobiles. Carbon monoxide is a health hazard because it can combine with the oxygen-carrying component of blood, preventing tissues from receiving sufficient oxygen. Lead has been linked with mental retardation in children. Vehicle emissions are now more strictly controlled than they once were and lead-free gasoline has virtually eliminated gasoline as a source of lead.

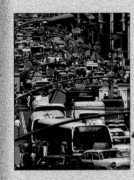

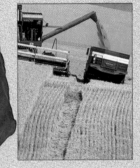

Chemicals in food

Using chemicals to fertilize crops or kill pests and using additives to preserve foods enables us to enjoy an abundant food supply. The Environmental Protection Agency monitors the toxicity of pesticides and the Food and Drug Administration monitors the use of additives. But the accumulation of pesticides in food may pose long-term health hazards, and some additives cause allergic reactions.

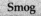

Smog

Smog, for the most part, is a result of the action of sunlight on nitrogen oxides and hydrocarbons released from automobile exhaust. Smog is highly irritating to the eyes and nose. The phenomenon has been particularly severe in large metropolitan areas.

CFCs

Chlorofluorocarbons (CFCs) are used in refrigeration and air-conditioning units and in the manufacture of insulation board for home construction. CFCs are thought to be responsible for erosion of stratospheric ozone, which blocks harmful ultraviolet rays from reaching the Earth. Higher ultraviolet levels increase the risk of skin cancer.

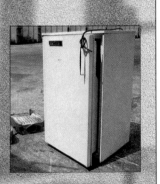

EFFECTS OF CLIMATE

Some regions with moderate climates are renowned as havens for elderly or chronically sick people. Moderate climates eliminate the need to dress for or adapt to extremes in temperature or variations in indoor heating and humidity. Certain illnesses also respond better to particular climates or may be aggravated by others. For example, people with chronic bronchitis, asthma, or rheumatoid arthritis do better in warm, dry climates than in damp, cold places. A person with chronic bronchitis is more likely to have an acute attack in winter. An asthma attack may be triggered by exercising in cold air.

Sunlight

A fair-skinned person living in a very sunny climate runs a much higher risk of skin cancer than a darker-skinned person. Incidence rates of skin cancer in Australia, for instance, are extremely high among people of European origin, but are negligible among native aborigines. It is especially important for fair-skinned people to protect themselves adequately from the sun and to examine their skin for early signs of skin cancer (see SKIN SELF-EXAMINATION on page 54). Some sunlight is necessary because it promotes the production of vitamin D in the skin. Children in some far northern communities in the Soviet Union are purposely exposed to artificial ultraviolet light during the dark winter months.

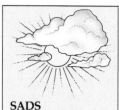

SADS

Some people appear to become depressed and anxious when sunlight hours are shorter, a phenomenon called seasonal affective disorder syndrome (SADS). Exposure to a light source that mimics natural sunlight seems to relieve symptoms in some people.

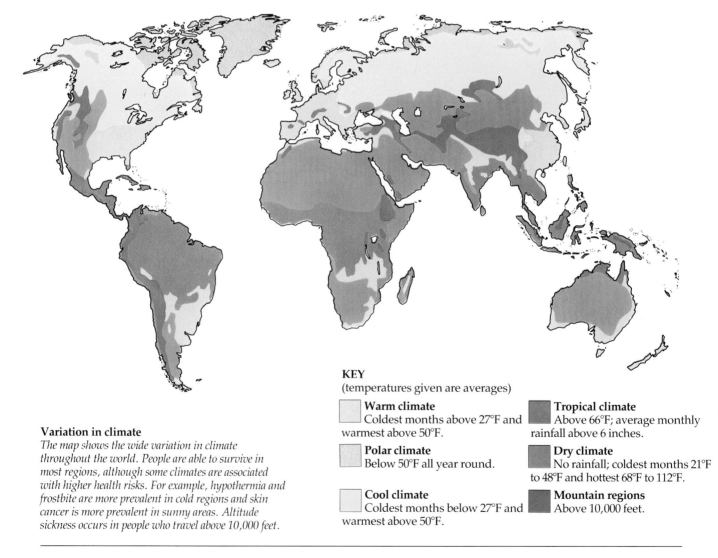

Variation in climate
The map shows the wide variation in climate throughout the world. People are able to survive in most regions, although some climates are associated with higher health risks. For example, hypothermia and frostbite are more prevalent in cold regions and skin cancer is more prevalent in sunny areas. Altitude sickness occurs in people who travel above 10,000 feet.

KEY
(temperatures given are averages)

Warm climate
Coldest months above 27°F and warmest above 50°F.

Polar climate
Below 50°F all year round.

Cool climate
Coldest months below 27°F and warmest above 50°F.

Tropical climate
Above 66°F; average monthly rainfall above 6 inches.

Dry climate
No rainfall; coldest months 21°F to 48°F and hottest 68°F to 112°F.

Mountain regions
Above 10,000 feet.

Altitude sickness

People who travel to altitudes higher than 10,000 feet may suffer from altitude sickness, especially if they ascend rapidly. Early symptoms include headache, nausea, loss of appetite, sleeplessness, and difficulty breathing. Anyone in whom symptoms develop should descend to a more comfortable level. Drug treatments are available, if required. Complete acclimatization to high altitudes takes about 6 weeks. In susceptible people or those who have heart or lung diseases, altitude sickness can develop into pulmonary or cerebral edema (an accumulation of fluid in the lungs or the brain). In these severe cases, descent to a lower altitude may be lifesaving.

Living high
The red blood cell counts of people who live at altitudes above 12,000 feet are higher than those of people who live at lower elevations. Higher numbers of red blood cells compensate for the decreased oxygen supply. The red blood cell counts of people who move to these high altitudes gradually increase to adapt to the new environment.

FOREIGN TRAVEL

Visiting foreign countries where the climate and standards of hygiene are different can cause ill health. If you have a medical condition, ask your doctor whether it is advisable for you to travel. At least 2 months before you leave, ask your doctor whether you need a vaccination or booster shot. The usual immunizations for adults, such as for tetanus and typhoid, should be up to date.

If you are traveling to a tropical or subtropical country, it is strongly recommended that you use an appropriate drug regimen and personal protective measures to avoid contracting malaria. Your doctor can advise you about the drugs that are most effective for the area you plan to visit. Take along mosquito netting and insect repellent, and wear clothing that covers most of your body. When you travel outside the US, Canada, Northern Europe, Australia, and New Zealand, food and drinking water can cause health problems. You can avoid problems by taking the following precautions:

◊ Boil all water, including any used for coffee or tea.
◊ Avoid eating shellfish, ice cream, egg dishes, raw or undercooked meat or fish, other uncooked foods, cream, and uncooked or unpeeled fruits and salads. A good rule is to eat fruits only if you have peeled them yourself and never buy food from street vendors.

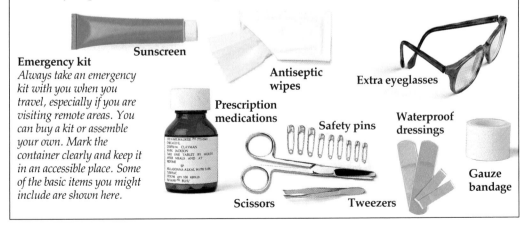

Emergency kit
Always take an emergency kit with you when you travel, especially if you are visiting remote areas. You can buy a kit or assemble your own. Mark the container clearly and keep it in an accessible place. Some of the basic items you might include are shown here.

Sunscreen

Antiseptic wipes

Extra eyeglasses

Prescription medications

Safety pins

Waterproof dressings

Scissors

Tweezers

Gauze bandage

BACKGROUND RADIATION

The natural ionizing radiation in the environment comes from two main sources – cosmic rays from outer space and radon gas that emanates mainly from the uranium that occurs everywhere in the Earth's crust. In the vast majority of cases, the amount of natural radiation is well within the limits currently regarded as safe. In some areas, particularly where granite rocks predominate, higher-than-average levels of radon gas may build up in houses. Simple, relatively accurate techniques are available to determine radon levels. High levels of radon can be reduced by increasing ventilation.

YOUR SEXUALITY

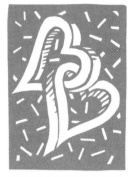

SEXUALITY IS A fundamental part of our physical and emotional lives. Sexual expression is a source of great pleasure and satisfaction for most men and women, yet celibacy – by circumstance or by preference – is also a normal variation. For many people, a good sex life is important but not always easy to maintain.

SEXUAL FREQUENCY

Many couples develop a pattern of sexual activity that is related to their work schedules, so that they can enjoy leisurely sexual intimacy. Of course they also can experience spontaneous expressions of desire. Illness, fatigue, or stress occasionally causes couples to alter their pattern of sexual activity. A dramatic, sustained reduction in a couple's usual level of sexual activity may indicate the possibility of a physical or emotional problem that needs attention.

Our inherited characteristics, our personality, our upbringing, our close affectionate relationships, and our first sexual experiences all affect our attitudes toward sex. They may enhance or hinder our ability to achieve sexual happiness. By becoming aware of the reasons for the satisfaction and dissatisfaction we may have, we can assess the attitudes and beliefs that enhance or interfere with our sexual health and habits.

IS YOUR SEX LIFE SATISFACTORY?

No one should ever expect his or her sex life to be perfect. Indeed, some experts believe that, while people may experience what they believe to be true love, the very nature of sexuality causes a tension that inevitably makes perfection impossible. Scientific studies of sexual

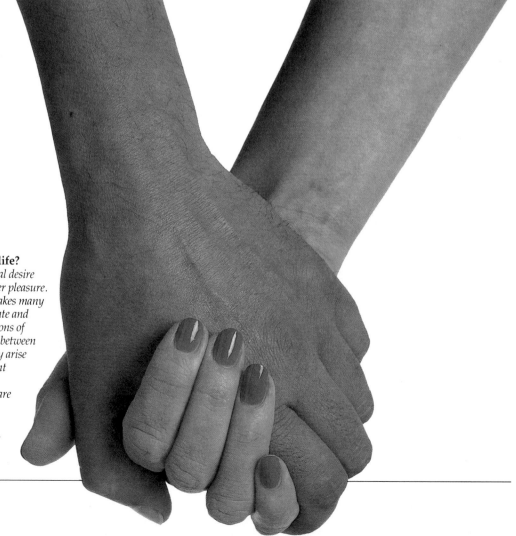

What makes a happy sex life?
The simplest answer is mutual desire and an effort to give each other pleasure. However, desire differs and takes many forms, ranging from passionate and direct to more subtle expressions of tenderness or understanding between partners. Problems frequently arise because partners have different ways of expressing desire. Differences are normal; they are neither good nor bad – just different – as are tastes in food. With mutual respect, partners can understand and accept each other.

happiness are increasingly showing that a "satisfactory" sex life is not as common as we might wish.

The reasons for dissatisfaction are many. For some people a simple lack of sex education may result in ignorance of normal sexual response. Others may have serious conflicts because of a violent experience such as early sexual abuse. Many problems between partners arise from unrealistically high expectations or misunderstandings about a partner's way of expressing desire. Sexual inhibitions related to upbringing may also be a source of problems.

Some psychologists believe that many people experience a conflict between the power of their biological sex drive and the learned inhibitions that seek to control that drive. Much sexual therapy today strives to help partners understand the forces that influence their sexual behavior and to negotiate changes so that the desires and needs of each may be equally considered. If the sexual behavior is unacceptable to society in general, the consequences of law infringe-ment must be openly discussed. A partner has the right to refuse to participate in any sexual activity if there is a serious clash of values. Equality and respect are important ingredients of a relationship.

Sexual problems – physical or psychological?

Difficulties in a relationship can cause problems with sexual functioning. The problems affecting men include impotence (inability to achieve or maintain an erection), premature ejaculation (ejaculating before or soon after penetration), or delayed or absent ejaculation. Women may experience painful intercourse, inability to have an orgasm, and vaginismus (in which the tightened vagina will not open enough to receive the penis in spite of adequate foreplay).

Although problems with sexual response are often linked with psychological factors, they are sometimes the result of disease, alcohol consumption, or use of other drugs. You should always check with your doctor about possible physical causes before seeking sex counseling.

SEXUAL ORIENTATION

An estimated 2 to 5 percent of men and women are homosexual. It is now generally recognized that homosexuality is a normal variation of sexual orientation and is not a psychological disorder. Research shows that attempts to change sexual orientation by therapeutic means are singularly unsuccessful. However, a young person should be encouraged to seek professional help to resolve emotional fears and problems. A homosexual person may seek counseling in order to come to terms with and accept his or her life situation.

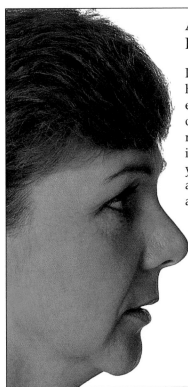
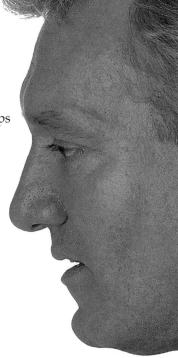

ARE YOUR SEXUAL EXPECTATIONS TOO HIGH?

People enter into sexual relationships with very high and often unattainable expectations. These expectations are partly based on romantic ideals of teenage years, media stereotypes, and the very real "high" of the initial attraction to a new, perhaps idealized, partner. No man is strong and capable, yet gentle at all times. He has weaknesses just like anyone else. No woman is sexually responsive around-the-clock and still a tireless co-earner and homemaker. She too has weaknesses. Relationships must be based on realistic expectations.

Communication is essential
Honest, open communication enhances closeness between partners and helps resolve the assumptions that are often at the root of conflict. Gestures, eye contact, smiles, laughter, phone calls, notes, and cards are among the forms of communication that many couples share. A "cold war" or an angry silence on the part of either partner is never a productive approach.

MONITOR YOUR SYMPTOMS
LOSS OF INTEREST IN SEX

Sex drive in men and women varies widely. Some people have a naturally low or high interest in sex, while others may have been affected by experiences in childhood or adolescence. If you and your partner have a satisfying sex life, frequency is irrelevant. However, a sudden loss of interest in sex may be the result of a treatable problem. Almost any illness can decrease your sex drive temporarily. Reactions to some medications may have the same effect. Emotional difficulties such as anger, anxiety, or depression are also very common causes.

KEY ♂ Men ♀ Women

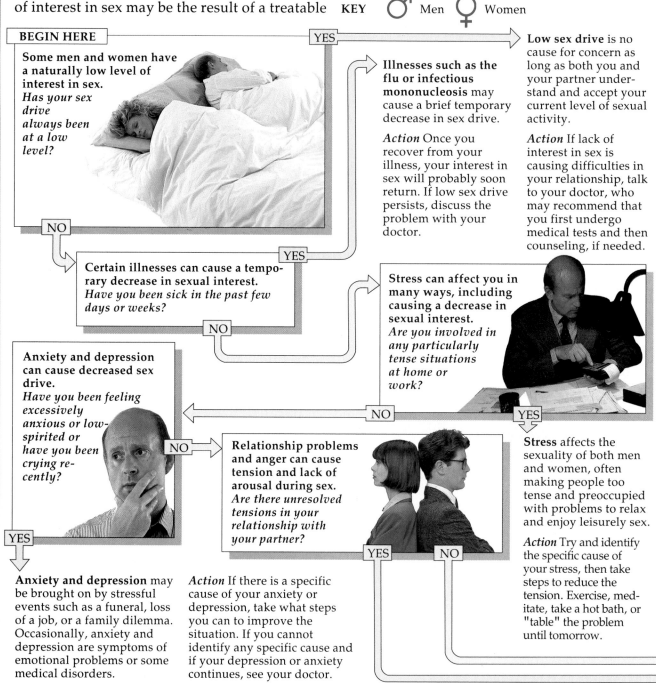

BEGIN HERE

Some men and women have a naturally low level of interest in sex.
Has your sex drive always been at a low level?

YES → **Low sex drive** is no cause for concern as long as both you and your partner understand and accept your current level of sexual activity.

Action If lack of interest in sex is causing difficulties in your relationship, talk to your doctor, who may recommend that you first undergo medical tests and then counseling, if needed.

Illnesses such as the flu or infectious mononucleosis may cause a brief temporary decrease in sex drive.

Action Once you recover from your illness, your interest in sex will probably soon return. If low sex drive persists, discuss the problem with your doctor.

NO

Certain illnesses can cause a temporary decrease in sexual interest.
Have you been sick in the past few days or weeks?

YES

NO

Stress can affect you in many ways, including causing a decrease in sexual interest.
Are you involved in any particularly tense situations at home or work?

Anxiety and depression can cause decreased sex drive.
Have you been feeling excessively anxious or low-spirited or have you been crying recently?

NO

NO

Relationship problems and anger can cause tension and lack of arousal during sex.
Are there unresolved tensions in your relationship with your partner?

YES

Stress affects the sexuality of both men and women, often making people too tense and preoccupied with problems to relax and enjoy leisurely sex.

Action Try and identify the specific cause of your stress, then take steps to reduce the tension. Exercise, meditate, take a hot bath, or "table" the problem until tomorrow.

YES

NO

YES

Anxiety and depression may be brought on by stressful events such as a funeral, loss of a job, or a family dilemma. Occasionally, anxiety and depression are symptoms of emotional problems or some medical disorders.

Action If there is a specific cause of your anxiety or depression, take what steps you can to improve the situation. If you cannot identify any specific cause and if your depression or anxiety continues, see your doctor.

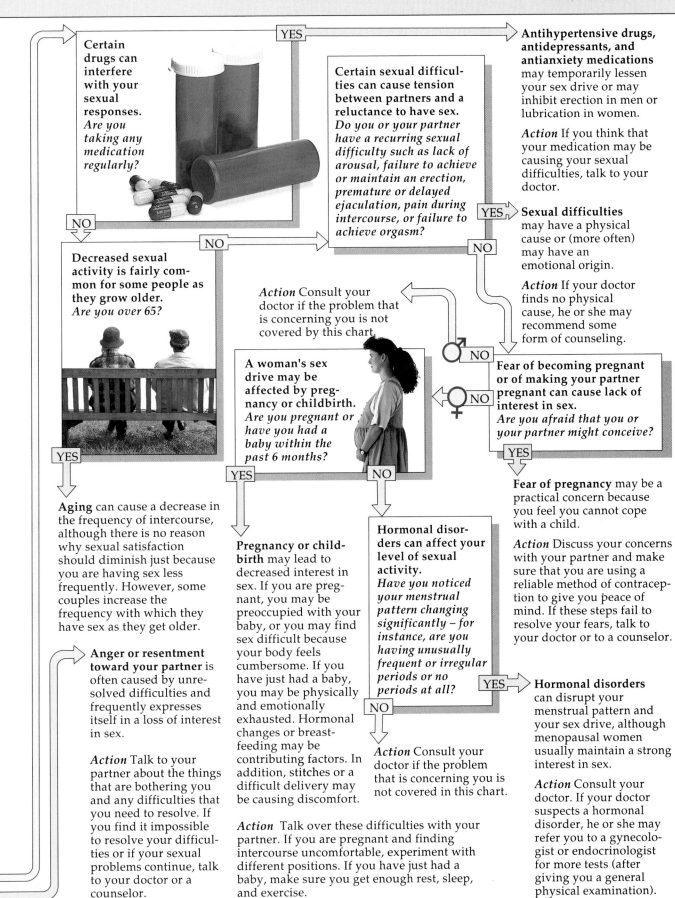

Certain drugs can interfere with your sexual responses. *Are you taking any medication regularly?*

YES → **Antihypertensive drugs, antidepressants, and antianxiety medications** may temporarily lessen your sex drive or may inhibit erection in men or lubrication in women.

Action If you think that your medication may be causing your sexual difficulties, talk to your doctor.

Certain sexual difficulties can cause tension between partners and a reluctance to have sex. *Do you or your partner have a recurring sexual difficulty such as lack of arousal, failure to achieve or maintain an erection, premature or delayed ejaculation, pain during intercourse, or failure to achieve orgasm?*

YES → **Sexual difficulties** may have a physical cause or (more often) may have an emotional origin.

Action If your doctor finds no physical cause, he or she may recommend some form of counseling.

NO

NO

Decreased sexual activity is fairly common for some people as they grow older. *Are you over 65?*

NO

Action Consult your doctor if the problem that is concerning you is not covered by this chart.

NO ♂

NO ♀

Fear of becoming pregnant or of making your partner pregnant can cause lack of interest in sex. *Are you afraid that you or your partner might conceive?*

A woman's sex drive may be affected by pregnancy or childbirth. *Are you pregnant or have you had a baby within the past 6 months?*

YES

YES → **Fear of pregnancy** may be a practical concern because you feel you cannot cope with a child.

Action Discuss your concerns with your partner and make sure that you are using a reliable method of contraception to give you peace of mind. If these steps fail to resolve your fears, talk to your doctor or to a counselor.

YES

Aging can cause a decrease in the frequency of intercourse, although there is no reason why sexual satisfaction should diminish just because you are having sex less frequently. However, some couples increase the frequency with which they have sex as they get older.

NO

Pregnancy or childbirth may lead to decreased interest in sex. If you are pregnant, you may be preoccupied with your baby, or you may find sex difficult because your body feels cumbersome. If you have just had a baby, you may be physically and emotionally exhausted. Hormonal changes or breastfeeding may be contributing factors. In addition, stitches or a difficult delivery may be causing discomfort.

Hormonal disorders can affect your level of sexual activity. *Have you noticed your menstrual pattern changing significantly – for instance, are you having unusually frequent or irregular periods or no periods at all?*

NO

Action Consult your doctor if the problem that is concerning you is not covered in this chart.

YES → **Hormonal disorders** can disrupt your menstrual pattern and your sex drive, although menopausal women usually maintain a strong interest in sex.

Action Consult your doctor. If your doctor suspects a hormonal disorder, he or she may refer you to a gynecologist or endocrinologist for more tests (after giving you a general physical examination).

Anger or resentment toward your partner is often caused by unresolved difficulties and frequently expresses itself in a loss of interest in sex.

Action Talk to your partner about the things that are bothering you and any difficulties that you need to resolve. If you find it impossible to resolve your difficulties or if your sexual problems continue, talk to your doctor or a counselor.

Action Talk over these difficulties with your partner. If you are pregnant and finding intercourse uncomfortable, experiment with different positions. If you have just had a baby, make sure you get enough rest, sleep, and exercise.

IMPROVING YOUR SEXUAL RELATIONSHIP

You can learn a great deal from reliable books about sexuality and sexual techniques, and you should never be embarrassed to consult such sources to improve your sexual satisfaction.

Neither should you hesitate to seek professional help for any problem that interferes with your enjoyment of sex. So much expertise is available today to help you deal with sex problems that it is only a question of looking for the correct resource. There is nothing unusual about having a sex problem, and you are not unusual if that problem is psychological because stress, fatigue, and conflict are part of everyone's life.

SEXUAL RESPONSES

To enjoy sex and to give your partner sexual enjoyment, it helps to understand male and female sexual responses. Intercourse falls into four main stages. The duration and intensity of each stage vary among individuals and with mood and age.

MEN

Arousal
The penis becomes erect in response to touch or thoughts.

Plateau
The penis reaches maximum size and the testicles elevate.

Orgasm
When a height of excitement is reached, semen is discharged from the penis, accompanied by intensely pleasurable sensations. There are also general contractions of all body muscles.

Resolution
The penis returns to its unstimulated stage, arousal disappears, and the person relaxes.

WOMEN

Arousal
Arousal occurs in response to physical touch or psychological stimulation. However, foreplay (such as kissing and touching) may be more important for women. The clitoris and vagina enlarge and the vaginal walls become moist. The nipples may become erect.

Plateau
All body muscles become tense.

Orgasm
The vagina contracts rhythmically several times, accompanied by intensely pleasurable sensations around the clitoris and the genital area. All the body muscles then contract a few times. Several orgasms in succession may occur.

Resolution
The breasts and genital organs gradually return to their previous state, arousal fades slowly, and the muscles throughout the body relax completely.

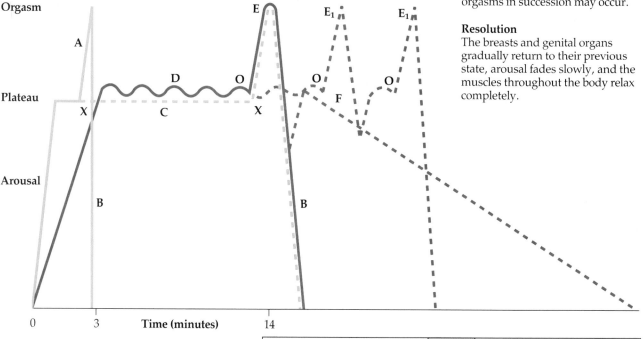

Male and female sexual response
The graph highlights the significant difference in timing of orgasm for men and women. The average man can reach orgasm in less than 3 minutes; the average woman reaches orgasm in approximately 14 minutes. An understanding of this difference in timing may help partners avoid unrealistic expectations about sexual performance or response. As the graph demonstrates, a man occasionally may sustain his erection until his partner reaches orgasm. A woman may experience one orgasm or multiple orgasms.

Men	KEY	Women
—— Average response		—— Average response
- - - Possible response		▪ ▪ ▪ Possible response
X Point of ejaculatory inevitability		**D** Prolonged plateau (arousal/lubrication)
A Average orgasm and ejaculation		**O** Point of orgasmic inevitability
B Softening and flaccidity		**E** Orgasm
C Sustained erection		**E₁** Multiple orgasm
		F Prolonged plateau/ no orgasm

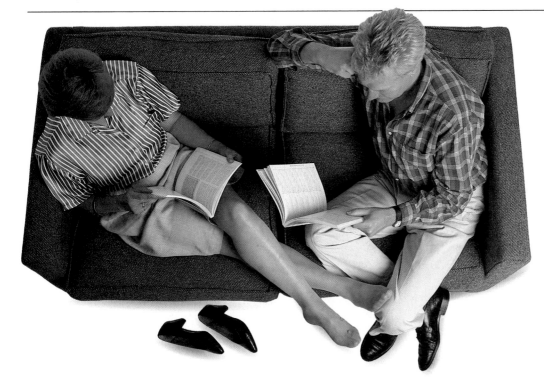

Learning about sex
Many excellent books on sexual technique and on relationship issues are available from bookstores or your local library. Do not hesitate to consult these sources. The best ones go beyond the mechanics of sexuality and deal in some detail with the all-important emotional aspects of sex.

Where can I get help?

You can seek help in several ways. You can consult your doctor, who will examine you to be certain there is no physical cause of the sex problem. Then, if necessary, you will be referred to a specialist. Alternatively, you can go individually or as a couple to a specialist of your choosing (perhaps a psychiatrist, marriage counselor, or sex therapist).

Whichever approach you take, it is important to remember that help is available today for any sexual problem you have. Sometimes treatment involves both partners for optimal outcome. There are times when a partner will say, "It's your problem. It has nothing to do with me!" However, there is seldom an "uninvolved" sexual partner. Both partners suffer when there is a problem and both partners gain when counseling restores a good relationship.

SEX AND THE AGE FACTOR

Studies show that men and women can physically enjoy sex well into their 80s and beyond. In later years arousal may be slower for both sexes. Erection is less firm and rapid (but does occur with longer, direct foreplay). Women after age 50 lubricate less easily and their vaginal walls lose elasticity. Both men and women may have a greater need for manual or oral stimulation. Understanding these factors can enrich a couple's ability to enjoy sex. The later years can provide the opportunity for partners to perfect their sexual skills and be more sensitive to each other's needs. Sex may become fulfilling in a different way than at earlier times in life.

The older couple
Research on sexuality carried out in the last decade has shown conclusively that men and women continue to experience sexual desire and fulfillment well into their 80s and beyond. In fact, after a woman has reached the menopause and pregnancy is not possible, both partners often find renewed interest and pleasure in their sexual relationship.

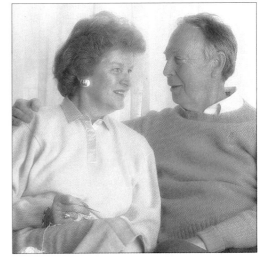

SEX AND PHYSICAL HEALTH

Having a healthy sex life means taking responsibility for ourselves and for our partners. If a person does not accept this responsibility, sex can result in the spread of sexually transmitted diseases or in an unwanted pregnancy.

Contraceptives: safety and effectiveness

Unwanted pregnancies usually can be prevented by the responsible use of contraception. A wide choice of methods is available, each differing in its effects and effectiveness, as well as its convenience. Apart from abstinence, sterilization is the most effective method of contraception. Two unreliable methods are periodic abstinence (the rhythm method) and male withdrawal during intercourse. Other choices of contraception are illustrated at right.

Caps and diaphragms
Several types of caps and diaphragms are available. They are harmless and very effective if used correctly with spermicidal jelly.

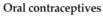

Condoms
Condoms are effective if used correctly and also provide protection against sexually transmitted diseases. Some types of lubricants may change the condom's effectiveness.

Sponges
Disposable foam sponges, impregnated with spermicide, come with loops for easy removal. The sponge must be left in position for at least 6 hours after intercourse.

Oral contraceptives
The oral contraceptive pill that contains progestogen and estrogen is highly effective. It can cause side effects such as headache, weight gain, or thrombosis (blood clots). Oral contraceptives also protect against ovarian and endometrial cancer. Progestogen-only pills have fewer side effects but are less effective contraceptives.

Spermicides
Used alone, spermicides are not very effective. But they provide additional protection with a condom, cervical cap, or diaphragm. Spermicides can cause allergic reactions.

Intrauterine devices (IUDs)
IUDs are effective but are linked with pelvic infection, ectopic pregnancy, and heavy or irregular bleeding. Most doctors limit use of IUDs to women in their late 30s and 40s who do not plan to have children.

CERVICAL (PAP) SMEAR

Cervical cancer can be cured if caught early enough. Every woman who has had sex should have a Pap smear at least once every 3 years, after two or three annual negative examinations. A woman who has had an abnormal smear in the past needs to have them more often, as her doctor recommends.

1 The woman lies on her back with her knees bent. She is asked to relax and allow her knees to fall apart. A speculum is inserted into the vaginal opening.

Speculum

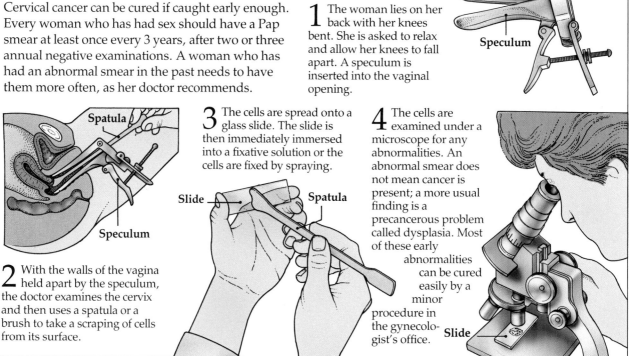

Spatula

Speculum

2 With the walls of the vagina held apart by the speculum, the doctor examines the cervix and then uses a spatula or a brush to take a scraping of cells from its surface.

3 The cells are spread onto a glass slide. The slide is then immediately immersed into a fixative solution or the cells are fixed by spraying.

Slide   **Spatula**

4 The cells are examined under a microscope for any abnormalities. An abnormal smear does not mean cancer is present; a more usual finding is a precancerous problem called dysplasia. Most of these early abnormalities can be cured easily by a minor procedure in the gynecologist's office. **Slide**

Are your sexual practices safe?

The fewer sexual partners you have, or have had, the less risk you have of sexually transmitted diseases, including infection with the AIDS virus. The safest behavior, other than total abstinence, is to have a monogamous relationship with an uninfected, monogamous partner. If you (or your partner) are having sex with more than one person, it is wise to have medical examinations on a regular basis.

If either you or your partner has, or may have, a sexually transmitted disease, you should always use a condom and spermicide. However, it is safest to avoid vaginal, oral, or anal sex, and any sexual practice that could involve contact with blood or broken skin. Avoid oral sex if either you or your partner has a cold sore around the mouth.

Most sexually transmitted diseases – and there are at least 25 of them – can be treated successfully. Untreated sexually transmitted diseases can cause serious medical problems. A woman can also pass a sexually transmitted disease to her baby before or during birth. If you have symptoms or signs of such a disease, consult your doctor immediately.

WARNING

The following symptoms and signs may indicate a sexually transmitted disease. However, remember that disease may be present without symptoms or signs.

- Penile discharge
- Abnormal vaginal discharge
- Sores, blisters, spots, or lumps on the genitals
- Irritation of the genitals
- Painful urination
- Passing urine more frequently than usual
- Pain during sexual intercourse
- Pain around the pelvic area
- Bleeding between periods
- Sore throat or a sore in or around the mouth
- Discharge, irritation, sores, or lumps around the anus

SEXUALLY TRANSMITTED DISEASES

The more common sexually transmitted diseases (STDs) are listed below.

Chlamydial infection was the most common STD in the US in 1990. As many as 4 million new cases occur each year. Untreated chlamydial infection can result in permanent damage to the reproductive organs. Chlamydial infections may not cause any symptoms or may cause a discharge or pelvic inflammatory disease in women or a penile discharge and irritation in men.

Genital herpes produces a painful, recurring rash on the genitals. It cannot be cured, but attacks tend to be less frequent and less severe as time goes by. Early treatment may reduce the severity of individual attacks.

Gonorrhea is one of the most common infectious diseases. Untreated, it may lead to sterility in men and women. A woman can pass the infection on to her baby during childbirth. Gonorrhea can also cause pelvic infections and arthritis.

Genital warts are painless growths that form on or around the genitals and are caused by the human papillomavirus. The virus has been shown to be a major cause of cervical cancer. Genital warts should be removed and a doctor should examine the affected area regularly.

Syphilis was on the decline for many years. However, its incidence is now rising, even in newborn babies. Untreated syphilis can lead to blindness, heart disease, or brain damage.

GENITAL SELF-EXAMINATION

Examine yourself carefully for redness, sores, blisters, or lumps on or around your genitals.

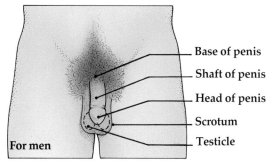

For men
- Base of penis
- Shaft of penis
- Head of penis
- Scrotum
- Testicle

1 Examine the head of your penis. If you are uncircumcised, pull back the foreskin to examine the head.

2 Examine the shaft of your penis, then examine the base. Separate the pubic hair to examine the skin underneath.

3 Examine your scrotum. Look at the skin and gently feel each testicle for lumps, swelling, or soreness.

Consult your doctor if you have any of the warning symptoms and signs listed above.

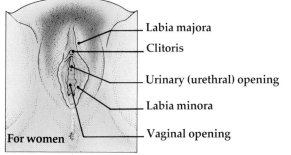

For women
- Labia majora
- Clitoris
- Urinary (urethral) opening
- Labia minora
- Vaginal opening

1 Examine the area covered by pubic hair, spreading the hair apart with your fingers.

2 Spread apart the outer vaginal lips (labia majora). Examine your clitoris, both sides of the inner lips (labia minora), and the areas of skin around the urinary opening (urethra) and the vaginal opening. A mirror makes the examination easier.

YOUR HABITS

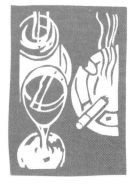

SINCE ANCIENT TIMES, people have turned to chemicals to help them relax, to stimulate them, or to alter their states of mind. Today, the most widely used legal substances of this kind are tobacco, alcohol, and caffeine. Although these substances may give us a temporary feeling of well-being, they all have harmful effects, especially alcohol and tobacco.

Most of us now know that smoking is damaging to health, but many smokers probably do not appreciate the implications of continuing their habit. Similarly, most drinkers know that overindulgence can have unpleasant effects, but they may not realize just how destructive excessive alcohol consumption can be to their physical and mental health. Studies of the possible damaging effects of caffeine are just beginning.

SMOKING

Although people have been using tobacco for centuries, the associated health risks were studied closely only as late as the 1950s. Since then, smoking has been identified as a major hazard, directly linked with cancer of the lung, oral cavity, esophagus, bladder, pancreas, and cervix, and with heart and circulatory disease, chronic bronchitis, emphysema, and fetal abnormalities.

In spite of these facts, the number of smokers worldwide has risen steadily

Teenage smoking
Most smokers start during their teenage years for reasons such as peer pressure or the desire to appear mature. Today, about 12 percent of 12 to 17 year olds smoke, and 35 percent of 18 to 25 year olds are smokers. Current figures show that 20 percent of high school senior girls are daily smokers, compared with 16 percent of high school senior boys.

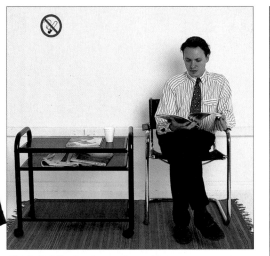

Social attitudes toward smoking
Smokers are facing increased pressure from non-smokers, largely because of the growing concern about the effects of passive smoking. Smoking is now restricted in many public facilities. Employers are also adopting policies to limit smoking in the workplace.

SMOKING DURING PREGNANCY

Smoking may harm your unborn baby. Pregnant smokers increase their risk of miscarriage and stillbirth and are more likely to have a premature or low-weight baby. Sudden infant death syndrome (crib death), respiratory problems, and some fetal abnormalities are more common among the infants of women who smoke.

SIGNS OF A SMOKING-RELATED PROBLEM

The symptoms described here are frequently, though not always, related to smoking. Whatever the cause of the symptoms, continuing to smoke will only aggravate them. Some smokers experience breathlessness, chest pain, and circulatory problems that improve quickly after they quit.

Breathlessness and wheezing
If you have difficulty breathing during exertion, your lung capacity has probably been impaired as a result of smoking. Shortness of breath and wheezing are two of the main symptoms of bronchitis and emphysema. These symptoms may progress to a crippling stage in some long-time smokers.

Digestive problems
If you frequently experience a burning sensation in your abdomen, nausea, vomiting, or episodes of belching, you may have a stomach ulcer or a duodenal ulcer, possibly induced by smoking.

Blood in urine
The presence of blood in the urine may be a symptom of bladder cancer and you should report it to your doctor immediately.

White or red patches in your mouth
Oral symptoms of this kind may be caused by precancerous changes and should be reported to your doctor or dentist immediately.

Coughing
If you have a persistent cough, you may have bronchitis. Chronic bronchitis develops in many smokers. Emphysema ultimately develops in many smokers who have bronchitis.

Chest pain
Chest pain brought on by exercise (angina) may be due to coronary heart disease. Chest pain is also common among bronchitis sufferers and sometimes indicates lung cancer.

Circulatory problems
If you experience frequent cramping pains in the lower part of your legs when you walk (intermittent claudication), your circulation may be impaired from smoking. Leg ulcers and, in extreme cases, gangrene of the lower part of the legs may eventually develop unless you stop smoking.

since the 1950s and so inevitably has the incidence of smoking-related diseases. However, many smokers in the US have quit. In 1964, 42 percent of the adult population smoked; in 1987, 29 percent smoked. At the same time, the gap between the numbers of male and female smokers has narrowed. Today, lung cancer has overtaken breast cancer as the most common fatal cancer in women. There has been an encouraging decrease in the percentage of adolescents who smoke, although the decline has been somewhat greater among young men than among young women.

Passive smoking

The dangers of tobacco smoke threaten not only the smoker who inhales it directly but also nonsmokers who breathe in air containing smoke. Some studies show that the secondary smoke that goes directly into the air from the burning tobacco contains more tar, nicotine, and carbon monoxide than the primary smoke that the smoker inhales. This secondary exposure, known as passive smoking, may cause irritation of the eyes, bronchi, lungs, nose, and sinuses in the nonsmoker. More seriously, regular passive smoking increases the risk of lung cancer. Infants and young children are particularly susceptible.

Quitting smoking

In order to give up smoking successfully, you must have a genuine desire to change your habits. No matter how long you have smoked, quitting will decrease your risk of a smoking-related disease. After about 15 nonsmoking years, the risks to the former smoker become almost equal to the risks to people who have never smoked.

When you stop smoking, overcoming your dependence on nicotine may be difficult. Your body will be cleared of nicotine within a few days of quitting, but the symptoms of withdrawal can last much longer. Part of your dependence on cigarettes is psychological. For some people, the smoking habit is influenced

QUITTING
Symptoms of nicotine withdrawal, such as headache, anxiety, and irritability, often weaken the resolve of a smoker who is trying to quit. You may wish to consult your doctor about the use of nicotine-containing chewing gum. This prescription product may help combat unpleasant withdrawal symptoms by slowing down the withdrawal process to some extent.

mainly by social or psychological factors, and avoiding situations that encourage smoking is important.

DRINKING ALCOHOL

Excessive alcohol consumption can lead to an increased risk of accidents and other consequences of alcohol intoxication and to addiction in the long run. In addition, alcohol can seriously damage your health.

Effects of alcohol

If you drink in moderation, you experience most of the pleasant effects of alcohol with the first drink or two. But feelings of increased mental and physical abilities are illusory. As more alcohol is consumed, mental and physical functions are increasingly impaired. A large amount of alcohol consumed over a short period of time can result in coma and even death. In the long run, heavy drinking leads to alcohol addiction and

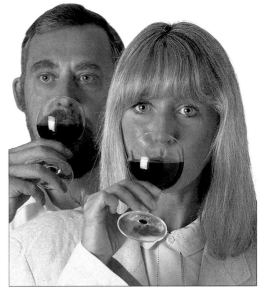

The effects of alcohol on men and women
Women have less tolerance to alcohol than men. Even taking lower weight into account, studies show that women feel the effects of alcohol sooner than men (after fewer drinks). This may be because of a difference in the degree to which women metabolize alcohol before it enters the bloodstream and because alcohol is removed from women's systems at a slower rate.

MONITOR YOUR CAFFEINE INTAKE

The caffeine contained in beverages such as tea, coffee, and cola acts as a stimulant that may increase alertness, improve thought processes, and help people with asthma breathe more freely. However, too high an intake may lead to anxiety or sleeplessness and unpleasant withdrawal symptoms when caffeine intake is restricted. Some people are particularly sensitive to caffeine and are better off avoiding it altogether.

Caffeine levels in milligrams (mg) per cup

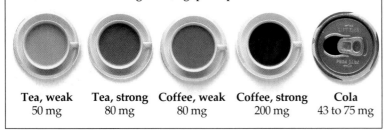

Tea, weak	Tea, strong	Coffee, weak	Coffee, strong	Cola
50 mg	80 mg	80 mg	200 mg	43 to 75 mg

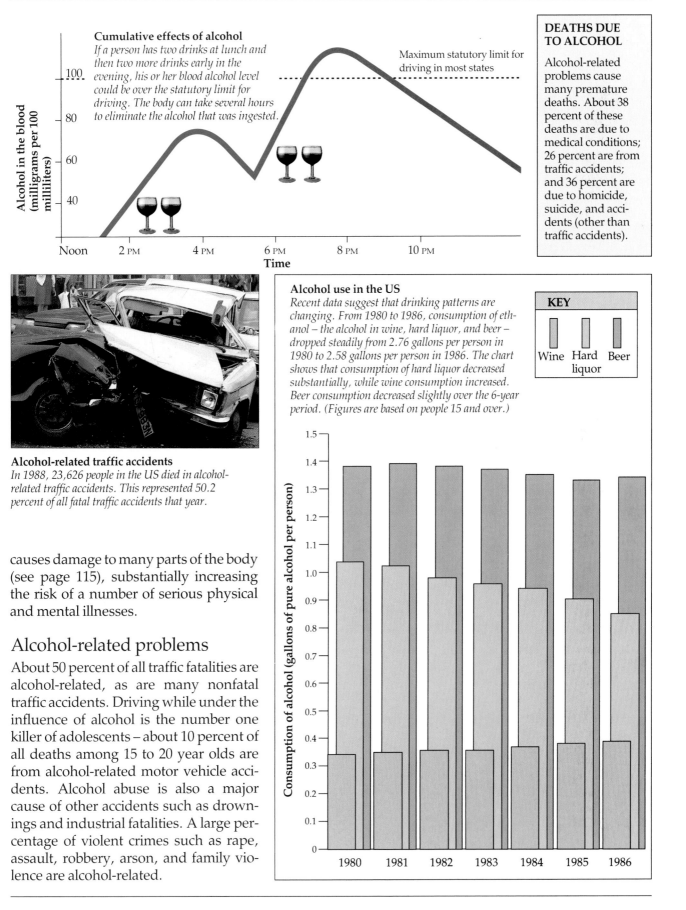

Cumulative effects of alcohol
If a person has two drinks at lunch and then two more drinks early in the evening, his or her blood alcohol level could be over the statutory limit for driving. The body can take several hours to eliminate the alcohol that was ingested.

Alcohol in the blood (milligrams per 100 milliliters)

100
80
60
40

Noon 2 PM 4 PM 6 PM 8 PM 10 PM

Time

Maximum statutory limit for driving in most states

DEATHS DUE TO ALCOHOL

Alcohol-related problems cause many premature deaths. About 38 percent of these deaths are due to medical conditions; 26 percent are from traffic accidents; and 36 percent are due to homicide, suicide, and accidents (other than traffic accidents).

Alcohol-related traffic accidents
In 1988, 23,626 people in the US died in alcohol-related traffic accidents. This represented 50.2 percent of all fatal traffic accidents that year.

Alcohol use in the US
Recent data suggest that drinking patterns are changing. From 1980 to 1986, consumption of ethanol – the alcohol in wine, hard liquor, and beer – dropped steadily from 2.76 gallons per person in 1980 to 2.58 gallons per person in 1986. The chart shows that consumption of hard liquor decreased substantially, while wine consumption increased. Beer consumption decreased slightly over the 6-year period. (Figures are based on people 15 and over.)

KEY

Wine Hard liquor Beer

Consumption of alcohol (gallons of pure alcohol per person)

1.5
1.4
1.3
1.2
1.1
1.0
0.9
0.8
0.7
0.6
0.5
0.4
0.3
0.2
0.1
0

1980 1981 1982 1983 1984 1985 1986

causes damage to many parts of the body (see page 115), substantially increasing the risk of a number of serious physical and mental illnesses.

Alcohol-related problems

About 50 percent of all traffic fatalities are alcohol-related, as are many nonfatal traffic accidents. Driving while under the influence of alcohol is the number one killer of adolescents – about 10 percent of all deaths among 15 to 20 year olds are from alcohol-related motor vehicle accidents. Alcohol abuse is also a major cause of other accidents such as drownings and industrial fatalities. A large percentage of violent crimes such as rape, assault, robbery, arson, and family violence are alcohol-related.

SHORT- AND LONG-TERM EFFECTS OF ALCOHOL

Having a drink can make you feel relaxed, confident, and sociable, but its effect on the brain is to impair mental functions. Heavy drinking can affect almost every organ of the body. In the long run, this can lead to many disorders. A habitual drinker acquires a tolerance to alcohol. This means that he or she gradually must drink more in order to achieve the same effect. The liver breaks down the alcohol at a faster rate, requiring the drinker to take in more in order to achieve the same level in the blood. At the same time, nerve cells in the brain become less and less responsive to a given amount of alcohol. Paradoxically, after years of drinking, many alcoholics experience a reduced tolerance.

WHAT HAPPENS WHEN YOU HAVE A DRINK?

Psychological effect of alcohol

Route of alcohol in the body

A glass of wine
Wine contains about 12 percent alcohol, but this amount can vary with the type and country of origin of the wine. Fortified wine such as sherry, port, and vermouth contains greater amounts of alcohol. The alcohol content of a wine is not necessarily related to its taste – a "robust" wine may contain less alcohol than a "delicate" wine.

Specific brain functions are affected
The first specific areas of the brain to be affected are the frontal lobes. The depression of these areas by alcohol reduces inhibitions and increases perception, self-confidence, and sociability, but clouds intellectual functions and judgment.

Alcohol reaches the brain
Within seconds, the alcohol reaches the brain and affects all areas. You experience a general feeling of relaxation because alcohol is a depressant.

An immediate psychological effect
The first taste of the drink may have an immediate relaxing effect. This may be partially a psychological reaction based on the memory that alcohol brings relaxation.

Alcohol enters the bloodstream
The alcohol reaches the stomach and intestines; new research shows that a significant amount of alcohol is metabolized in the stomach. The alcohol is absorbed into the bloodstream and is carried to every tissue in the body.

Alcohol is broken down and excreted
The liver gradually breaks down the alcohol. A small amount of alcohol passes unchanged into the urine.

DRINKS CONTAINING THE SAME AMOUNTS OF ALCOHOL

The drinks illustrated below, in the amounts indicated, contain approximately the same amounts of alcohol. However, different wines, beers, and liquors can vary widely in their alcohol content. Check the percentage indicated on the bottle.

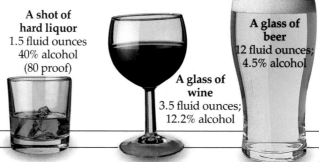

A shot of hard liquor
1.5 fluid ounces
40% alcohol
(80 proof)

A glass of wine
3.5 fluid ounces;
12.2% alcohol

A glass of beer
12 fluid ounces;
4.5% alcohol

HOW THE BODY IS AFFECTED BY LONG-TERM, HEAVY DRINKING

The brain
Brain damage from repeated, excessive consumption of alcohol can cause intellectual deterioration, depression, memory loss, and eventually dementia.

The mouth, throat, and esophagus
The risk of cancer of the mouth, throat, and esophagus is increased. Blood vessels in the esophagus may enlarge and bleed easily.

The skin
The skin may deteriorate because of poor eating habits. Damage to blood vessels may cause permanent flushing.

Fat
Weight gain due to an increase in fat cells often occurs because alcohol is loaded with calories. One drink rarely contains less than 100 kilocalories.

The liver
There is a serious risk of cirrhosis (see below left), hepatitis (inflammation), fatty liver, and liver cancer.

The heart and circulation
Excessive alcohol use can lead to heart disease, high blood pressure, anemia, and disorders of blood clotting.

The digestive system
Excessive drinking can lead to stomach ulcers, gastritis (inflammation of the stomach), and inflammation of the pancreas. Long-standing inflammation of the pancreas can cause a loss of digestive enzymes, leading to chronic diarrhea. Alcoholics often have an inadequate diet, resulting in poor nutrition.

A cirrhotic liver
Permanent scarring of the liver is caused by heavy drinking.

The nerves
Excessive drinking can temporarily or permanently impair nerve function.

The reproductive system
Heavy drinking can lead to infertility in both sexes, menstrual problems in women, and impotence in men. Effects on sex hormones in men may also enlarge the breasts and shrink the testicles.

FETAL ALCOHOL SYNDROME

Drinking even small amounts of alcohol during pregnancy can damage the fetus. Fetal alcohol syndrome is the third leading cause of birth defects. Abnormalities may include retarded growth and physical deformities, cleft lip and palate, heart defects, and mental retardation.

115

CASE HISTORY
A CONCERNED DRINKER

ELAINE HAD BEEN WORKING for several years in an advertising agency. After work she usually joined some of her coworkers at a nearby bar and often drank throughout the evening. She drank even more heavily at weekend parties. Recently, she became concerned about an ache under her right rib, nausea, loss of appetite, and a yellow tint to her eyes. She made an appointment with her doctor.

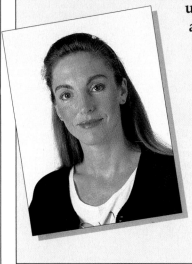

PERSONAL DETAILS
Name Elaine Barnhart
Age 34
Occupation Advertising manager
Family Elaine's father was an alcoholic; he died at 57. Her mother is well.

MEDICAL BACKGROUND

Until now, Elaine has not had any serious illnesses. She always intends to eat a more balanced diet and get some exercise, but the pace of her work schedule seems to interfere.

THE CONSULTATION

Elaine's doctor takes a detailed medical history. Upon questioning Elaine, he discovers that, in addition to the abdominal pain, she has been sleeping badly. He notes that she is slightly overweight. When Elaine takes a deep breath, her doctor feels the slightly rounded, tender edge of her liver flip under his fingers. He also detects some evidence of jaundice (yellowing of the skin and eyes caused by damage to the liver). He is fairly certain that Elaine's problems are the results of excessive alcohol consumption. He arranges for some blood tests and he suggests that she keep an honest record of her drinking over the next week.

THE DIAGNOSIS

When the doctor sees Elaine again, he tells her that the tests confirm that she has ALCOHOLIC HEPATITIS (inflammation of the liver, with some cell damage) and fatty infiltration of the liver. He tells Elaine that her condition is completely reversible at this time. He cautions her that she is in a high-risk category for the development of cirrhosis (an irreversible liver disease), not only because of the large quantity of alcohol she consumes, but because women have a lower

Monitoring alcohol intake
Elaine's doctor suggests that she keep a record of all the drinks she has in a week, noting whom she was with and where she was at the time. The record reveals, to her dismay, that she has consumed 35 drinks in the past week.

tolerance for alcohol than men. The doctor tells Elaine that she may be addicted to alcohol. He strongly advises her to stop drinking alcohol and to get treatment from an addiction specialist who has experience with alcoholism problems. He recommends to Elaine that she rest and eat a nourishing diet during her recovery from hepatitis.

THE FOLLOW-UP

Within a couple of months, Elaine's symptoms are gone. She has met with the addiction specialist who has counseled her about her habits; he has referred her to a support group for people with drinking problems. Elaine is resolutely avoiding the after-work drinking scene, and she has joined a dance class that meets twice a week. Now that she realizes her predisposition to alcoholic hepatitis and alcohol addiction, she understands the importance of avoiding alcohol and learning to deal with the situations that tempt her to indulge.

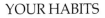

Alcohol addiction

Alcoholism – alcohol addiction – is a preventable and treatable disease. Current estimates suggest that there are about 12 to 15 million alcoholics in the US. If you or someone close to you drinks large amounts of alcohol, you should be aware of signs indicating that addiction may have developed. Your doctor can obtain information by taking a medical history, performing a physical examination, and interpreting the results of blood tests of liver function, which detect damage caused by heavy drinking.

The sooner alcoholism is treated, the better the chances are of a complete recovery. But a long-term problem drinker can also get effective treatment. A number of organizations offer active support groups (see right).

GETTING HELP

Call your local Alcoholics Anonymous (AA) for help with recovery from alcoholism. You will find the number in your telephone book under "Alcohol" or "Alcoholism." For information on alcohol problems, talk to your doctor and call the National Council on Alcoholism and Drug Dependence (NCADD) at 1-800-NCA-CALL.

DO YOU HAVE A PROBLEM WITH ALCOHOL?

Below is a test to help you review the role of alcohol in your life. Answer each question either "yes" or "no."

1. Do you occasionally drink heavily after a disappointment or an argument or when you have had a hard day at work?

2. Do you drink more when you have problems or feel under pressure?

3. Were you ever unable to remember part of an evening when you had been drinking, even though your friends say you didn't pass out?

4. When drinking with other people, do you try to conceal having a few extra drinks?

5. Do you sometimes feel uncomfortable if alcohol is not available?

6. Do you sometimes feel a little guilty about your drinking?

7. Do you often want to continue drinking after your friends say they've had enough?

8. When you are sober, do you often regret things you did or said while drinking?

9. Have you tried switching to another type of alcohol or following different programs to control your drinking?

10. Have you broken promises you made to yourself about controlling or cutting down on your drinking?

11. Have you tried to change your drinking habits by changing jobs or relocating?

12. Do you try to avoid family or close friends while you are drinking?

13. Are you having financial and work problems because of your drinking?

14. Do you sometimes have the "shakes" in the morning and find that it helps to have a drink?

15. Have you recently noticed that you can't drink as much as you once could?

16. Do you sometimes stay drunk for several days at a time?

17. Do you get terribly frightened after you have been drinking heavily?

Any "yes" answer indicates a possible alcohol problem. More than one "yes" means that you are probably addicted to or becoming addicted to alcohol. You should seek help.

ASK YOUR DOCTOR
YOUR HABITS

Q Why do alcoholic drinks cause a hangover, and how can you prevent or cure one?

A All alcoholic drinks cause you to lose more fluid than usual in urine and the resulting dehydration is the cause of most hangovers. The metabolic breakdown products of alcohol are toxic and also contribute to a hangover. Brandy, red wine, and bourbon contain a higher level of substances (called congeners) that, by their effect upon the brain, usually produce particularly severe hangovers. Drinking as much water as you can after drinking alcohol can help to counteract the effects of dehydration. The "hair of the dog" method could reflect alcoholism.

Q Should I give up smoking by stopping suddenly or by gradually cutting back?

A You will probably have a better chance of quitting smoking if you stop completely. Brief use of nicotine gum to help you withdraw from nicotine may help, particularly when used in addition to a behavior modification program. Individual counseling is also helpful.

Q Would switching to cigars or a pipe be healthier for me than smoking cigarettes?

A No. Unlike most cigar or pipe smokers, who do not usually consciously inhale the smoke, cigarette smokers who switch tend to inhale, and their risk of lung cancer may be increased. This is because the inhaled cigar and pipe tobacco smoke has a higher content of carcinogenic tar and nicotine.

CHAPTER FIVE

HEALTH AND AGING

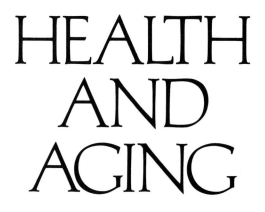

INTRODUCTION

PACING YOURSELF

COPING
WITH CHANGE

SPECIAL
HEALTH PROBLEMS

ILLIONS OF PEOPLE today live into their 80s and 90s free of serious medical conditions, particularly if they have monitored their health throughout their lives. In this chapter, we try to dispel some of the myths associated with growing older. Although some deterioration of body systems occurs as a result of aging, many of these changes need not significantly affect an older person's ability to function. Of course, some illnesses are more common among the elderly and we highlight those of major importance. Most of these problems are not inevitable.

We begin by looking at the aging process – the physical and mental changes that occur – and we tell you how you can help slow these processes by maintaining a healthy way of life. We discuss some of the challenging aspects of aging, such as the risk of depression and the likelihood of having to cope with bereavement. We examine the social changes that advancing age brings and discuss how you can cope effectively with these transitions. We stress the opportunities for growth and self-fulfillment that the later years offer. In addition, we focus on the importance of having a positive mental attitude and remaining active and involved.

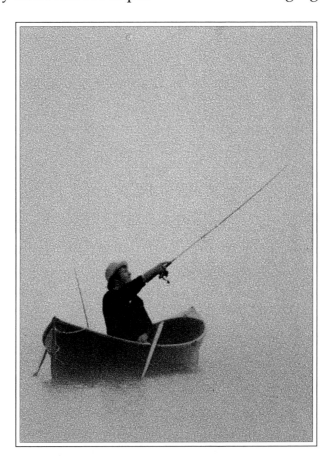

As we grow older it is more important than ever to watch our health closely because we are susceptible to more health problems. We summarize those aspects of general health that may require special attention in the older person, such as nutrition, vision, hearing, oral health, and foot care. The risk of accidental injury, especially from falls and burns, increases with advancing age. Most accidents occur in the home, and we outline the steps you can take to make your home safe for an older person.

The three major killers of people over 65 years of age are heart disease, cancer, and cerebrovascular disease (stroke), but you can decrease your risk of dying of one of these disorders by making sure you have regular checkups, by continuing to perform self-examinations, and by being aware of possible symptoms. The short-term memory loss that occurs with age is not a cause for concern; however, sometimes progressive memory loss is a sign of an underlying psychological or medical problem. We discuss the possibility of dementia, emphasizing the importance of proper evaluation. Finally, we include current information about drugs and point out the common problems associated with medication in older people.

PACING YOURSELF

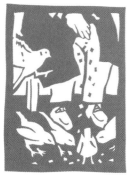

MEN AND WOMEN who have kept their bodies in good condition show few signs of physical and mental slowing until well into their 60s. At 60, your physical strength can be 80 percent of what it was at 25; your muscles will remain strong as long as they are used. Many people in their 70s are capable of running marathons or playing vigorous games such as tennis, while also retaining skill and authority in their daily work.

In the latter third of your life, your physical and mental abilities may begin to change. If you have always been very active you may need to make only moderate adjustments in your physical activities. You may need to learn new ways to improve your memory. Or you may simply need to compensate by making lists, keeping a daily calendar, or writing down details that you must handle.

PHYSICAL CHANGES

Even for a person in perfect health, age brings physical changes. Most changes are related to a progressive loss of elastic tissues, which leads to wrinkling of the skin and loss of flexibility in joints and muscles. Cellular structure breaks down somewhat too, so that the skin becomes

THE AGING PROCESS

Brain and nervous system
Loss of nerve cells reduces the ability to memorize or to learn new skills. Reaction times are slower.

Heart and circulation
The heart becomes less efficient, reducing exercise tolerance. Arteries degenerate, causing poor circulation and higher blood pressure.

Lungs
Loss of elasticity makes breathing less efficient.

Liver
The liver becomes less efficient in processing toxins in the blood.

Joints
Pressure on discs reduces height. Joints lose mobility.

Muscles
There is loss of muscle bulk and strength.

Loss of bone density
With age, bones become progressively less dense and weaker, a condition known as osteoporosis. The dense structure of young bone can be seen in the illustration at right. By contrast, the older, osteoporotic bone at far right shows many spaces where protein and calcium have been lost.

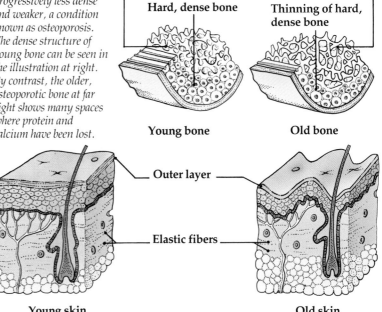

Soft, spongy bone

Hard, dense bone

Thinning of soft, spongy bone

Thinning of hard, dense bone

Young bone

Old bone

Outer layer

Elastic fibers

Young skin

Old skin

Skin changes
Young skin has a thick outer layer, and the deeper layers have many collagen fibers, which make the skin elastic. With age, the outer skin layer thins and becomes more prone to injury. The number of elastic fibers in the deeper layers decreases, causing the skin to become wrinkled and loose.

thinner and the muscles lose some of their bulk. Osteoporosis, the thinning of bone, is another inevitable characteristic of aging. These changes in the basic structures of the body make older people more susceptible to injuries – muscles tear and bones fracture more easily. Injuries heal more slowly as well.

MENTAL CHANGES

The physical changes of aging are paralleled by changes in mental function. Learning and retaining facts become more difficult as we get older, and memory becomes less reliable. The positive side of aging is that an older person has accumulated experience (sometimes defined as learning from mistakes), which is why many cultures revere their elders for their wisdom.

SLOWING DOWN THE AGING PROCESS

Research offers convincing evidence that your behavior can influence the rate at which both physical and mental changes occur. "Use it or lose it" is valid advice. The more bones and muscles are used, the better their condition. Regular exercise slows the pace of osteoporosis and muscle thinning. Your sexual function also will benefit from continued activity. The same concept applies to mental activities. Keep stimulating your intellect by reading new books, taking classes, traveling, meeting new people – even working crossword puzzles.

Another important means of moderating the rate at which you age is to avoid abusing your body. Heavy drinking causes brain damage and accelerates dementia; tobacco smoking is also damaging. Eat a healthy diet and exercise regularly. The key to enjoying a healthy old age is to recognize that growing older is inevitable but that you can slow down the aging process by setting sensible physical and mental goals.

JOINT REPLACEMENT

The replacement of diseased or damaged joints by artificial substitutes of metal or plastic is a remarkable achievement of high-technology medicine. Joint replacement is widely used to benefit people with degenerative arthritis. It is also done for people with severe cases of rheumatoid arthritis.

Today, most artificial joints are cemented in place. Because some (especially hip) joints have shown a tendency to loosen with time, surgeons are currently evaluating a range of cementless prostheses. These are designed so that bone grows into spaces in the metal, forming a strong, natural bond.

What joints can be replaced?

Full mobility has been restored to hundreds of thousands of people who have had arthritic hip joints replaced. Other joints are replaced less frequently and with varying degrees of success. However, artificial knees, shoulders, ankles, and elbows are all available. Even finger joints can be replaced.

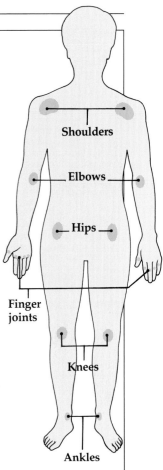

Shoulders

Elbows

Hips

Finger joints

Knees

Ankles

NEW KNEE JOINTS

Replacing an arthritic knee joint with artificial parts can relieve pain and restore some degree of mobility. A knee prosthesis cannot restore the full range of motion, but researchers continue to develop designs that will provide even greater mobility.

Femur

Patella

Tibia

Fibula

Knee joint prosthesis
An artificial knee joint consists of two major parts, which are fitted onto the ends of the tibia and femur after they have been cut, shaped, and drilled.

Femoral component

Tibial component

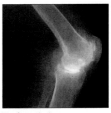

Before joint replacement
This X-ray of an arthritic knee joint shows severe wear and tear on bone and cartilage.

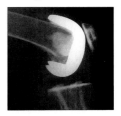

After joint replacement
In this X-ray, the two components of the artificial knee joint are shown in place.

COPING WITH CHANGE

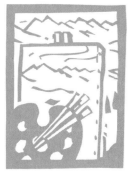

CHANGE — VOLUNTARY OR INVOLUNTARY — can be difficult at any age. As we grow older, we face largely involuntary changes directly related to aging that may be unlike problems we confronted earlier in life. If we continue to stimulate our minds and our senses, we can (given reasonable physical health) remain vital and able to cope with challenges and enjoy the benefits of later life.

Positive attitude
The key to staying mentally fit as we age is continued stimulation. It is never too late to study a new subject or learn a new skill. Later life, which often brings increased leisure time, may be the opportunity to try something you have always wanted to do.

As we grow older, we need to realistically assess changes in our lives. Our children grow up and leave home. We may reduce our previous job responsibilities or stop working completely. With advancing age, the possibility that a loved one may die increases. Coping with change and loss can be extremely difficult. It is important that we stay alert to the signs that may indicate someone is suffering from intolerable stress or an overintense reaction to grief.

MENTAL ATTITUDE

Mental attitude is an extremely important element in the process of aging. If we believe that we can go on functioning successfully, although perhaps not as quickly as we did when we were younger, then we can continue to learn and mature and enjoy life fully. Increasing withdrawal, deterioration, and pessimism are not inevitable aspects of old age.

Short-term memory does deteriorate slightly with age and our reactions slow. However, as people get older, they trade speed for precision and accuracy, and there is in fact very little noticeable difference in overall performance.

Healthy older people usually keep up a level of social activity very similar to that of their earlier years. Evidence shows that continued social activity is important to physical and emotional

PLANNING FOR RETIREMENT

Retirement brings important changes in a person's life – changes that require major readjustments. You should begin planning for retirement well ahead of the expected date. You may wish to enroll in a course that prepares you for retirement. You may also find it helpful to consider the following interrelated aspects of your life:

♦ **Income and assets** Talk to a financial adviser about establishing a budget for your retirement.

♦ **Continuation of work activities** Consider part-time or volunteer work so you will not feel isolated.

♦ **Social support** Make sure you have a network of friends and relatives you can call on in times of need.

♦ **Leisure** Find out about local social activities. Get involved before you retire.

♦ **Where to live** You may wish to stay where you have been living and where you already have friends. If you intend to move, learn about your new location. Important considerations include leisure facilities and transportation.

each year. You may also find it useful to write down more specific, short-term goals, perhaps for the next month.

Interact with younger people

Both young and old sometimes have difficulty communicating with each other. Younger people may respond to an elderly person with a type of fear – not knowing how to cope with attitudes or disabilities that they have not yet encountered. At the same time, the older person may not appreciate the changes that have occurred in the culture, thus increasing the lack of communication. However, everyone benefits from the opportunity to get to know members of another generation. Younger people can prompt seniors to look at things in new ways. An older person can pass on cultural values, knowledge, and experi-

well-being. We need to continue stimulating our minds with new experiences. Learning a new language or a new skill, such as photography, can provide this stimulation. Meeting new people is also satisfying. If you are retired you might consider becoming involved in community activities or taking classes that involve different circles of friends.

Have a sense of purpose

Motivation may diminish slightly with age because the pressure of your responsibilities may decrease. However, mental energy derives largely from expectations and goals and you may need to refocus your attention on a new set of priorities. You may find the following exercise helpful.

Try writing down all the things you might want to accomplish or experience within the next 3 to 5 years. They can be social, career, or artistic goals or new places you want to see or people you want to meet. Refine the list several times until it accurately reflects your most deeply felt desires. Strive to accomplish at least one of the items on this list

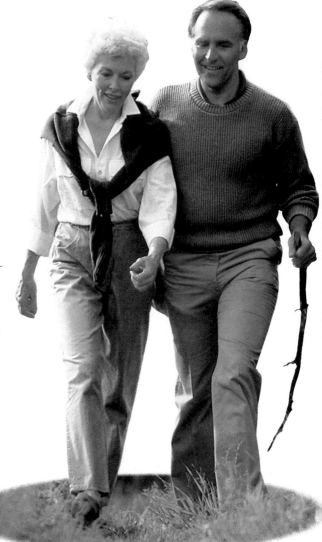

Exercise and independence
Regular physical exercise – such as walking a mile four times a week – benefits your mind and your body. It increases your alertness, leading to faster reaction times. It tends to counteract depression, making you feel more optimistic and raising your self-esteem. Research also shows that people who exercise regularly in later life remain functionally independent longer than less active people.

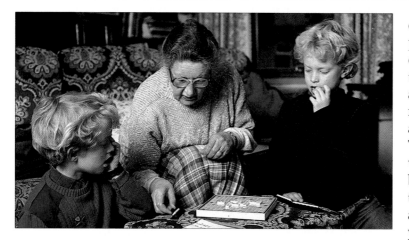

ence to a younger person, as well as provide services that contribute to his or her own sense of usefulness.

DEPRESSION

Depression may be the most prevalent psychological disorder at any age. Tolerance for stress may be lower among people in their later years than in younger age groups because of the frequency and intensity of stressful life events that an older adult may experience. Of course, depression does not always have a psychological cause. Many disorders to which the older person is susceptible and the use of some prescribed drugs can precipitate depression. Almost any illness or stress that strikes a person at an emotionally vulnerable time can provoke depression. The symptoms of an illness may force the aging person to recognize that his or her physical and mental capacities are deteriorating.

Recognizing depression
Most instances of depression are mild and are highly responsive to short-term therapy. Depression can affect anyone, so it is important to recognize its symptoms. The signs of depression in an older person are similar to those that occur at any age. Sleeping too little or too much, loss of appetite, and fatigue are common signs of depression. A depressed person may lose interest in life, have trouble concentrating, and lose his or her sexual

Coping with loss
Finding companionship and maintaining family ties is an important means of coping with the losses that come with old age. Depression is common among older people and is frequently caused by some form of loss, such as bereavement, retirement, or loss of mobility. A sense of isolation may be one aspect of depression. For example, the death of a spouse at a time in life when children are grown and are living away from home may intensify the loss.

SLEEP AND AGING

As people age, they need less sleep at night but may nap during the day. Depression, anxiety, and lack of exercise are among the factors that can affect sleep patterns. A person who is depressed tends to wake in the early morning. Anxiety can prevent a person from falling asleep at night. Getting enough exercise and establishing a regular sleep/wake routine helps.

desire. All of these signs need not be present; any one sign may indicate depression. Such signs are often mistakenly presumed to be consequences of aging. Depressed older adults may dismiss their low level of interest, fatigue, and withdrawal as "normal for their age." There is no reason for them to feel this way. People of all ages can savor life and be optimistic about the future. Effective treatment for depression is readily available. Never hesitate to seek the help of your family doctor if you or any older person you know shows a marked change in mood, habits, or behavior.

Successful aging
In 1985, there were 28 million people over the age of 65 in the US. Some estimates indicate that, by the year 2030, that figure will be as large as 65 million. Advances in medical science have helped older members of society a great deal. Recent research has focused on the factors that contribute to successful aging – that is, growing older with minimal physical disability and with an ongoing sense of well-being. Findings suggest that personal control and social support are highly influential factors. When an older person is in control of events in his or her life, health and quality of life are significantly better. Similarly, a strong, supportive social network of family and friends has a positive effect on longevity and emotional well-being.

BEREAVEMENT

As people grow older, they must cope at some time with the death of someone close. The loss of a loved one may trigger a very intense emotional grief reaction, which can threaten mental and physical health. An extreme grief reaction is a major risk factor for suicide, particularly for an older, socially isolated man. Research has shown that recent bereavement is associated with an increased susceptibility to disease and to death from a variety of disorders. If death comes un-expectedly, the person left behind may have difficulty coping with the abrupt loss. The grieving person copes with the loss in stages (see STAGES OF BEREAVE-MENT at left). Anyone who has lost a loved one experiences some or all of these stages. The survivor needs to work through these feelings in order to come to terms with the loss. Of course, no two people react in exactly the same way. The stages may overlap, the order may vary, and some stages may be omitted altogether. The period that each lasts is also variable, but you can expect the entire grieving process to last 1 to 2 years.

Helping the bereaved

Immediately after a death has occurred, you can offer practical help such as assistance with funeral arrangements and preparation of food. But the most important contribution you can make is just being available to listen. Above all, do not be driven away by the person's anger and depression, even though these emotions may be difficult for you to deal with. A grieving person needs continuous support for many months. Finally, you should take any threat of suicide seriously and help the bereaved person get professional help immediately.

STAGES OF BEREAVEMENT

♦ **Shock and denial** This stage features a kind of emotional numbness and difficulty accepting what has happened.
♦ **Anger toward oneself or others** During this stage, the grieving person feels angry and resentful that a cherished person has been taken away. Feelings of guilt are also common.
♦ **Searching** At this point, the person yearns to recover what has been lost and keeps looking and hoping for the return of the loved one. Hallucinations involving the dead person are not uncommon.
♦ **Mental depression and associated guilt** When anger has gone, the grieving person may become uninterested in life. Life may not seem worth living. Guilt – feeling somehow responsible for the person's death – may contribute to the depression.
♦ **Acceptance** The survivor must pass through this essential stage in order to return to a normal life. This stage usually involves reminiscing about the dead person and gradually coming to terms with the loss.

PROLONGED OR EXCESSIVE GRIEF

If you experience any of the following extreme reactions to bereavement, you may wish to seek professional advice:

♦ Excessively high levels of anxiety
♦ Not being able to get through any stage of the grieving process
♦ Extreme feelings of guilt
♦ Inability to cope with daily activities

Emotional support
A bereaved person needs someone who will simply "be there." Be ready to listen patiently and give the person an opportunity to talk about his or her loss. Active response is not always necessary.

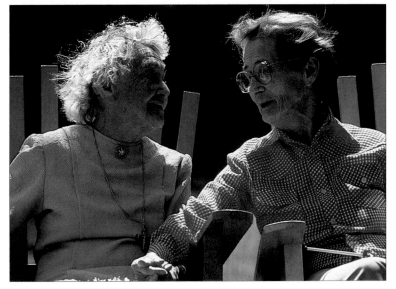

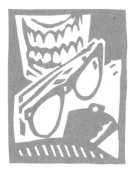

SPECIAL HEALTH PROBLEMS

A S OUR POPULATION AGES, older men and women realize that many of the problems often associated with old age are manageable. A wide range of information, services, and products are available to help an older person with his or her specific physical, psychological, and social needs.

It is important to continue to monitor your health as you get older or to watch for health problems in an older relative and identify signs and symptoms that may require medical attention. It is always preferable for an older person to take responsibility for his or her own health as a manifestation of personal independence and self-sufficiency.

MONITORING COMMON PROBLEMS

The health considerations that are important throughout your lifetime – diet, exercise, and awareness of changes in your own body – are equally or more important in later life.

Eating habits

People tend to eat less as they get older, in part because they have become more sedentary. If you have become less active, it is appropriate to reduce your food consumption in order to avoid excessive weight gain. Better still, if your health permits, you can maintain or even increase your level of exercise.

A healthy diet
Make sure your diet contains plenty of fresh vegetables and fruit, whole-grain bread, a moderate amount of protein, and a small amount of fat. Many cookbooks are available today that provide interesting yet healthy recipes. Some specialized cookbooks are written for people with specific conditions such as heart disease.

For some people, dietary inadequacy becomes a problem. They may eat a sufficient quantity of food but variety and balance are lacking. An older person may have difficulty getting to a grocery store or preparing food. Such difficulties may lead to vitamin deficiencies or general malnutrition, which, in turn, increases susceptibility to illness. An unbalanced diet that is low in fiber is a factor in the development of constipation.

At any age your diet should be balanced and should include an adequate amount of fluids. Weigh yourself regularly. If you lose or gain a few pounds, monitor the change to see if it continues. If it does, see your doctor.

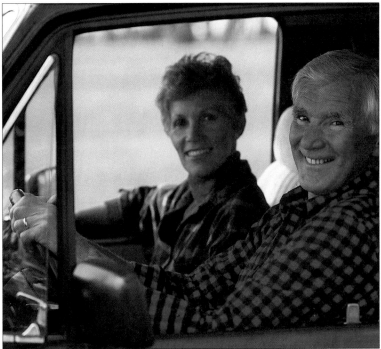

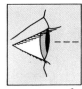

Getting enough fluids
In temperate climates, you should drink at least 4 or 5 pints of fluids a day. This habit helps you avoid problems such as dehydration and constipation.

Vision

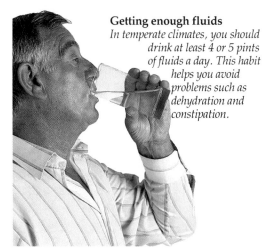

Focusing ability usually becomes impaired with increasing age because the eye lenses lose their elasticity and their ability to accommodate (see page 32). It is important to have regular professional eye checkups, whether or not you already wear glasses (see page 17). Eye diseases often impair the vision of older people. Glaucoma (raised internal pressure in the eye), cataract (clouding of the internal lens of the eye), and macular degeneration (loss of vision in the center of the field of vision) are more common among the elderly population, so it is important to watch for signs of these diseases (see pages 33 and 34). Cataract removal and lens implants are now straightforward, highly successful procedures that have restored lost vision to many people. Permanent damage to the eyes from glaucoma or macular degeneration can be prevented or at least halted by early diagnosis and treatment.

Hearing

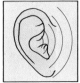

With age, hearing ability – particularly sensitivity to higher-frequency sounds – may be impaired. Understanding speech may become increasingly difficult. You can use the suggestions and tests on page 36 to check your hearing. An older person you know may have an undiagnosed hearing loss. He or she may be greatly helped by the use of a hearing aid (see page 37). It is a common misconception to assume that a person is losing his or her memory or becoming withdrawn when in fact hearing loss is the problem. If you already use a hearing aid, you should continue to have periodic professional checkups to ensure that the hearing aid is functioning correctly and adequately.

Should you drive?
To be a safe driver, you must be able to see well – with or without glasses. Wear your glasses if you need them for driving. Your neck movements should be fairly unrestricted. You must be capable of operating all the controls on the car. Don't drive if you are taking medication that may make you drowsy or dizzy, or if you are subject to fainting or uncontrolled seizures. Ask your doctor for advice. Your reactions tend to become slower as you get older, so adjust your driving speed accordingly. Also, try to avoid driving in unusually heavy traffic or after dark.

Feet

Healthy feet are essential to mobility. Foot disorders are very common and particularly dangerous in older people. The feet are complicated structures, full of tiny joints and muscles that can stiffen with age. Ensure that you have a good pair of well-fitting shoes, and avoid spending too much time in soft shoes or slippers that do not adequately support your feet.

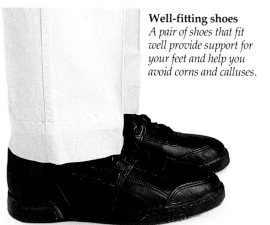

Well-fitting shoes
A pair of shoes that fit well provide support for your feet and help you avoid corns and calluses.

Overly tight or loose shoes cause pressure or rubbing on prominent points on your feet, which may lead to corns and aggravate bunions. It also becomes harder to keep your nails in good shape as you get older. Wash your feet every day and, to avoid ingrown toenails (see page 46), don't cut your nails too short.

Teeth and dentures

Some people maintain a full set of healthy teeth until an advanced age, but many people lose their teeth because of dental problems that started earlier in life. If you wear dentures it is important that they fit well. Loose dentures may impair your ability to eat and speak. Dentures that rub may cause discomfort and irritation of the gums. Signs of gum disease include bad breath, sore gums, discoloration, or discharges from the base of the teeth. If you have any of these symptoms, consult your dentist immediately.

HYPOTHERMIA

Hypothermia (dangerously low body temperature) may occur in sick, elderly people who live in inadequately heated homes in cold climates. Older people gradually lose their sensitivity to cold and cannot always respond to a cold environment. Symptoms of hypothermia include pallor, drowsiness, listlessness, confusion, and facial puffiness. The person's pulse may be unusually low, and the skin may feel cold. If you are concerned that someone's body temperature is dangerously low, seek medical help immediately.

FLU SHOTS AND PNEUMONIA SHOTS

Influenza, a viral infection popularly known as the flu, can be particularly debilitating or even fatal to an older person. An annual flu shot in the fall is recommended if you are over 65, especially if you have a chronic illness such as heart disease, bronchitis, emphysema, or diabetes. The vaccination offers 6 to 8 months of protection for 60 to 90 percent of those who receive it. The vaccine is changed annually to contain strains of the viruses that experts believe are most likely to spread.

For protection against pneumonia – once a common killer of the aged – you can now get a once-in-a-lifetime vaccination. The shot contains most, if not all, of the strains of pneumococcal bacteria, which are among the causes of pneumonia. Some authorities recommend this immunization for everyone over 65. The shot is particularly important for people who have chronic respiratory disease.

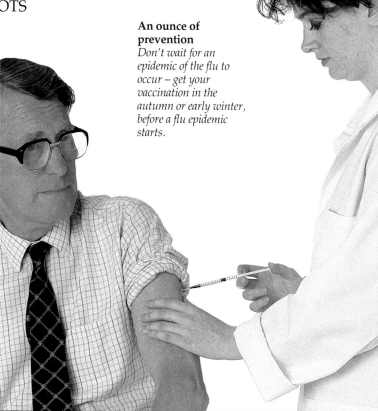

An ounce of prevention
Don't wait for an epidemic of the flu to occur – get your vaccination in the autumn or early winter, before a flu epidemic starts.

CASE HISTORY
DETERIORATING VISION

REBECCA IS AN **established painter. For months she has been concerned about her vision. Recently, two clients refused to pay for their paintings and a customer suggested that her work was not up to its usual high standards. Rebecca became seriously worried and decided to consult an ophthalmologist.**

PERSONAL DETAILS
Name Rebecca Diaz-Ortega
Age 72
Occupation Professional painter
Family No history of significant disease.

MEDICAL BACKGROUND
Rebecca's medical history is unremarkable except that, at age 67, she had a hip replacement. She has been undergoing hormone replacement therapy for several years.

THE CONSULTATION
Rebecca tells the ophthalmologist that she doesn't wear glasses when she paints, but that she does wear her glasses, which have a strong prescription, when she reads. Recently she has had some problems reading. She also says that her perception of color has been changing. The world looks less blue than before and yellows and reds seem accentuated. Vision testing shows that the acuity in each of Rebecca's eyes is reduced to 20/60 with glasses on, and a stronger prescription does not improve her vision.

The ophthalmologist uses drops to dilate Rebecca's pupils and examines the internal structures of her eyes with an illuminated microscope. He checks the pressure in her eyes and then examines her retinas with an ophthalmoscope.

THE DIAGNOSIS
Rebecca's retinas are healthy and the internal pressure in both eyes is normal. However, both of her internal crystalline lenses have gradually suffered from protein changes that have altered the transparency of the lenses. One of the lenses has a large, cloudy, opaque area. The ophthalmologist explains that this is a common form of CATARACT and reassures her that a simple operation will restore her vision and color perception to normal. Rebecca accepts his diagnosis and explanation of her symptoms, but declines treatment because she is uncomfortable with the idea of having an eye operation.

Several months later she returns because she can no longer work and is now having increased difficulty reading. The ophthalmologist explains the procedure thoroughly and the operation is set for the following week.

THE TREATMENT
The operation is performed (with the aid of a local anesthetic) in the ophthalmologist's operating suite. The lens of Rebecca's right eye is removed from its capsule and replaced with a tiny, optically perfect, plastic lens that has been tailored to her vision requirements. When the bandage is removed, she is ecstatic to find that her vision has improved dramatically. Three months later, because the protein changes in her left eye still alter her vision, she returns eagerly to the hospital to have her left lens replaced.

THE OUTLOOK
Rebecca has perfect distance vision but needs glasses for painting and reading. She returns to her work with renewed vigor and reestablishes her base of clients.

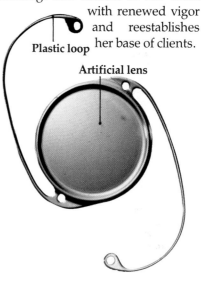

Plastic loop

Artificial lens

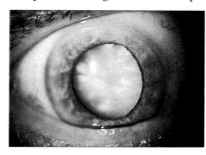

Treatment for cataract
The photograph above shows the appearance of an advanced cataract before treatment. Treatment consists of removing the cloudy internal lens of the eye and replacing it with a tiny plastic lens as shown at right.

IS YOUR HOME SAFE?

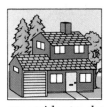

Accidents are a major cause of injury and death among all age groups. However, the risk of certain types of accidents increases with age. Falls, car accidents, choking on food or some object, and burns or asphyxiation as a result of house fires are the most common accidents among elderly people. Most accidents involving older people occur at home, and attention to home safety can greatly reduce the risks. If an older person moves to a new home, the loss of familiarity with the environment may trigger an accident. However, the major factors in accidents among the elderly are age-related physical infirmities and medical problems. Less acute hearing and sight and slower reflexes make it harder to detect and avoid hazards. Medical disorders that affect mobility or cause sudden loss of consciousness obviously increase the risk of accidental injury and possible serious complications for an older person.

Falls and their complications

Falls are the leading cause of accidental death at home among people over 65 years old. Because of their more brittle bones, older people can easily fracture their hips, wrists, or even spines. More than one third of the falls that occur among people over 75 result in such fractures. Elderly women are particularly at risk of fractures because osteoporosis causes them to experience greater loss of bone substance than men. Elderly women also fall more frequently than elderly men, for reasons that are not clear.

Falls may also have a serious psychological impact on an aging person. A fall experience (or the fear of falling) may cause a previously active person to unnecessarily decrease his or her activities.

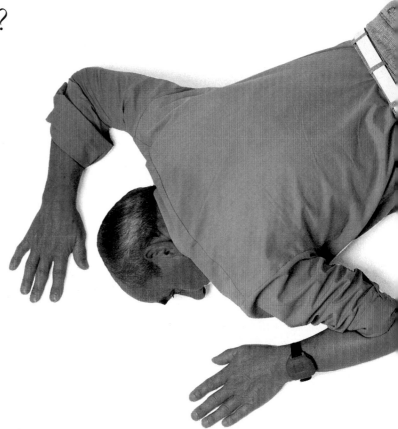

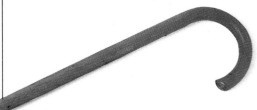

Hazards at floor level
The majority of falls occur at floor level rather than from a height. Check your home for the hazards illustrated at right. To reduce the likelihood of a fall, consider removing rugs and mats from your home and carpeting slippery floor surfaces to reduce the risk of injury.

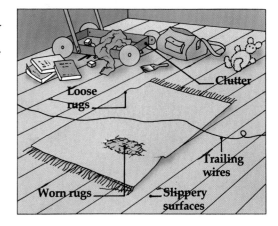

Loose rugs

Clutter

Trailing wires

Worn rugs

Slippery surfaces

Stairs
Many falls among elderly people occur on stairs. Check your stairs regularly for the hazards shown at right. Some older people choose to move to a single-level house.

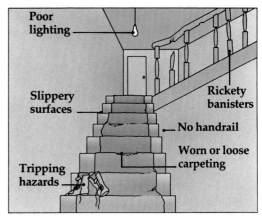

Poor lighting

Slippery surfaces

Rickety banisters

No handrail

Worn or loose carpeting

Tripping hazards

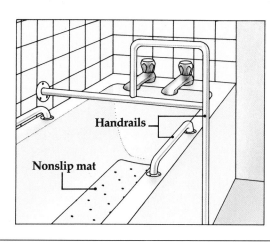

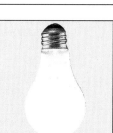

Should you be using an alarm?
If you do fall, the outcome is likely to be much more serious if you lie unattended for more than an hour, particularly in a cold environment. Pneumonia or hypothermia may develop. An alarm device may be lifesaving if you live alone. Most devices consist of a necklace or bracelet with a button that you can activate to send a distress signal by telephone.

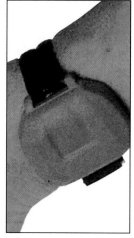

WARNING

Frequent falls are usually a symptom of a medical problem, particularly if the falls occur because you lose consciousness. If you have been falling regularly, with or without loss of consciousness, consult a doctor at once. The factors listed below may be involved:

♦ A problem with vision, hearing, or balance
♦ Drug therapy involving sedatives or antihypertensive medication
♦ Poor mobility from arthritis or parkinsonism
♦ Any condition that causes you to lose consciousness, such as epilepsy, irregularities of heart rhythm, or a decrease in blood pressure when you stand up

HOW BRIGHT IS YOUR HOME?

Having adequate lighting in your home is an important way to reduce the risk of accidents. Older people require plenty of light in all rooms but especially around more dangerous areas such as stairs or hallways. Use the brightest bulbs possible in your light fixtures. It is wise to install night-lights in all hallways and rooms or to have timers or remote-control switches for lights so that you never need to walk across a dark room to turn on a light.

Burns and accidents associated with fire
Home deaths and injuries from burns or scalding or from accidents associated with fire are highest among people 65 years and older. You can reduce the risks by taking precautions such as having gas and electrical systems serviced regularly and by installing fire extinguishers and smoke detectors throughout your home. If you have a fireplace, make sure you use a fireplace screen, and do not sit too close to the fire.

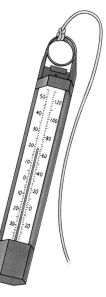

Controlling water temperature
Sensitivity to temperature declines with age so older people sometimes find it difficult to judge water temperature. To avoid being scalded, you can use a special thermometer such as the one shown at left to test water temperature. You can also fill a tub or sink with cold water before adding hot water to help guard against injury. Thermostats on water heaters should always be set appropriately.

Safety in the bathroom
If you have stiff joints you may experience pain when you try to lower yourself into the bathtub. If you are unsteady, you may fall while trying to get in or out of the tub. Equipment such as that shown at left may give you more peace of mind when you take a bath.

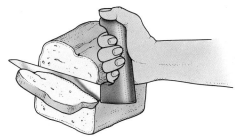

Handrails

Nonslip mat

Kitchen safety
Specially designed kitchen implements can protect an older person against cuts and burns. This knife has a large, angled handle and can be used with minimal pressure. A person with arthritis can handle such a knife easily and safely.

THE THREE MAJOR CAUSES OF DEATH

The three main causes of death among people over the age of 65 are heart disease, cancer, and cerebrovascular disease (stroke). For signs and symptoms of heart disease and cancer, see pages 48 to 56.

Cerebrovascular disease may interrupt blood flow in the small vessels supplying the brain. It can be caused by high blood pressure, atherosclerosis (in which fatty deposits narrow the arteries), blood clots, or hemorrhage. Paralysis or multi-infarct dementia may result (see page 136).

A transient ischemic attack (see below) temporarily decreases the blood supply to the brain and can be a sign of cerebrovascular disease. Treatment can prevent or delay progression of the disease. It is important to be tested for high blood pressure and be treated if necessary (see page 55).

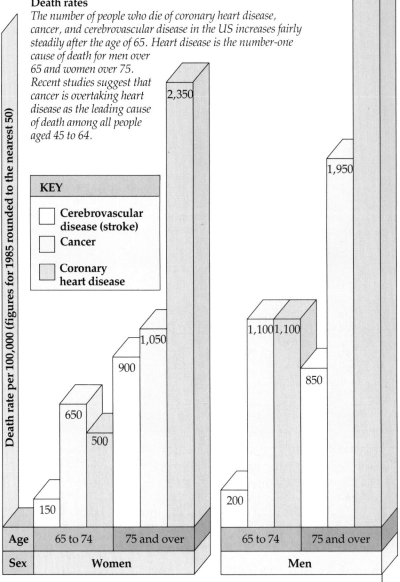

Death rates

The number of people who die of coronary heart disease, cancer, and cerebrovascular disease in the US increases fairly steadily after the age of 65. Heart disease is the number-one cause of death for men over 65 and women over 75. Recent studies suggest that cancer is overtaking heart disease as the leading cause of death among all people aged 45 to 64.

Death rate per 100,000 (figures for 1985 rounded to the nearest 50)

KEY

☐ Cerebrovascular disease (stroke)
☐ Cancer
☐ Coronary heart disease

Age	65 to 74	75 and over	65 to 74	75 and over
Sex	Women		Men	

Women 65 to 74: 150, 650, 500
Women 75 and over: 900, 1,050, 2,350
Men 65 to 74: 200, 1,100, 1,100
Men 75 and over: 850, 1,950, 3,150

WARNING

Get medical attention at once if you experience one or more of the following signs or symptoms, lasting from a few minutes to several hours. You may be having a transient ischemic attack.

♦ Loss or disturbance of vision in one of your eyes
♦ Partial paralysis on one side
♦ Loss of feeling on one side
♦ Speech impairment
♦ Dizziness
♦ Immobility or unsteadiness
♦ Weakness or numbness
♦ Loss of memory

INCONTINENCE

The involuntary and unwanted passing of urine, or sometimes feces, is something no one likes to discuss. As a result, it is one of the most undertreated medical conditions. Incontinence is more common among older people than among the young, and affects women more often than men. You should always report incontinence to your doctor. Once your doctor has determined the cause – and this is usually possible – he or she can treat the condition appropriately. Even if the condition cannot be cured, advice about special clothing or urine-collecting devices can be helpful.

Urinary incontinence

Causes of urinary incontinence include weakened sphincter muscles (which allow control over the emptying of the bladder), urinary infections, obstruction of the outflow from the bladder, and dementia (which reduces the awareness of, or the ability to express, the need to urinate). For some women, childbirth

URINARY INCONTINENCE

Stress incontinence
Stress incontinence is common among women who have had children. This condition causes the release of a small amount of urine while coughing, sneezing, and laughing, during strenuous activity, or when performing weight-bearing exercise. Pelvic floor exercises and hormone treatment may help resolve the problem.

WOMAN

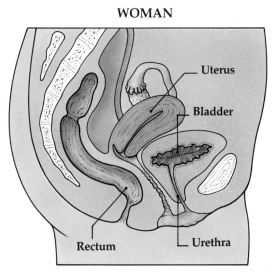

Urge incontinence
Urge incontinence may be caused by a bladder infection, kidney stones, or a diuretic medication. When internal pressure in the bladder reaches a certain level, the person has a strong urge to urinate, followed by an involuntary contraction and emptying of the bladder. Treatment with medication is not very satisfactory. Elimination of the cause is the best means of treatment.

The irritable bladder
An irritable bladder may be caused by a urinary tract infection or stress. The bladder muscle contracts intermittently, pushing out a small amount of urine and causing an intense desire to urinate.

Overflow incontinence
Overflow incontinence is a result of obstruction by an enlarged prostate gland. The bladder fills up completely and remains full and then, at regular intervals, releases a small involuntary "overflow" of urine. Prior to removal of the prostate, draining the bladder with a catheter can relieve the condition.

MAN

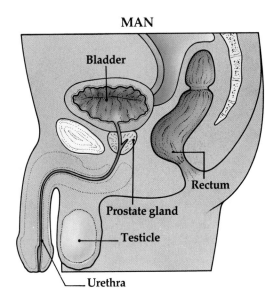

may weaken the pelvic floor muscles, which can contribute to incontinence. Some diseases that cause brain or spinal cord damage also affect bladder control. Medications, anxiety, psychological stress, anger, and frustration are other contributing factors.

Fecal incontinence

Ironically, fecal incontinence is often caused by severe constipation. The feces become hardened and fill the lower part of the rectum. As a result, the less-formed and liquid stool above the rectum is involuntarily forced out when the person strains to move the bowels. This condition is called fecal impaction and the fecal material must be broken up manually and flushed out with enemas.

Fecal incontinence may be caused by a serious neurological disorder (such as paralysis, multiple sclerosis, or dementia) and may be reduced by the regular use of enemas.

HEALTH ASSESSMENT FOR OLDER PEOPLE

Doctors now recognize that it is important to assess whether an older person is functioning as independently as his or her physical and emotional status permits. Current assessments seek to determine whether the individual has the self-confidence, bolstered by social and financial support, that he or she needs. Awareness is increasing among health care professionals of the importance of this kind of overall functional assessment. The resources are now more commonly available to provide social support, physical therapy, and other health-related services to older people.

MONITOR YOUR SYMPTOMS
FORGETFULNESS AND CONFUSION

People of every age have days when they have trouble remembering important things or are easily confused. Generally this problem arises when an individual is temporarily under stress or fatigued. Mild forgetfulness is also a common sign of aging. However, if you suddenly notice or, more likely, others question whether you are becoming unusually forgetful or confused, there may be an underlying medical problem that needs assessment.

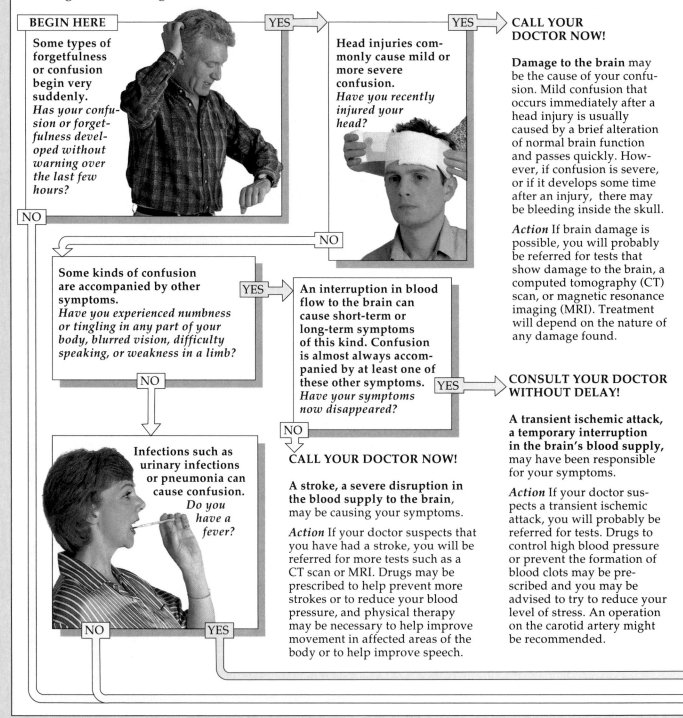

BEGIN HERE

Some types of forgetfulness or confusion begin very suddenly.
Has your confusion or forgetfulness developed without warning over the last few hours?

Head injuries commonly cause mild or more severe confusion.
Have you recently injured your head?

Some kinds of confusion are accompanied by other symptoms.
Have you experienced numbness or tingling in any part of your body, blurred vision, difficulty speaking, or weakness in a limb?

An interruption in blood flow to the brain can cause short-term or long-term symptoms of this kind. Confusion is almost always accompanied by at least one of these other symptoms.
Have your symptoms now disappeared?

Infections such as urinary infections or pneumonia can cause confusion.
Do you have a fever?

CALL YOUR DOCTOR NOW!

Damage to the brain may be the cause of your confusion. Mild confusion that occurs immediately after a head injury is usually caused by a brief alteration of normal brain function and passes quickly. However, if confusion is severe, or if it develops some time after an injury, there may be bleeding inside the skull.

Action If brain damage is possible, you will probably be referred for tests that show damage to the brain, a computed tomography (CT) scan, or magnetic resonance imaging (MRI). Treatment will depend on the nature of any damage found.

CONSULT YOUR DOCTOR WITHOUT DELAY!

A transient ischemic attack, a temporary interruption in the brain's blood supply, may have been responsible for your symptoms.

Action If your doctor suspects a transient ischemic attack, you will probably be referred for tests. Drugs to control high blood pressure or prevent the formation of blood clots may be prescribed and you may be advised to try to reduce your level of stress. An operation on the carotid artery might be recommended.

CALL YOUR DOCTOR NOW!

A stroke, a severe disruption in the blood supply to the brain, may be causing your symptoms.

Action If your doctor suspects that you have had a stroke, you will be referred for more tests such as a CT scan or MRI. Drugs may be prescribed to help prevent more strokes or to reduce your blood pressure, and physical therapy may be necessary to help improve movement in affected areas of the body or to help improve speech.

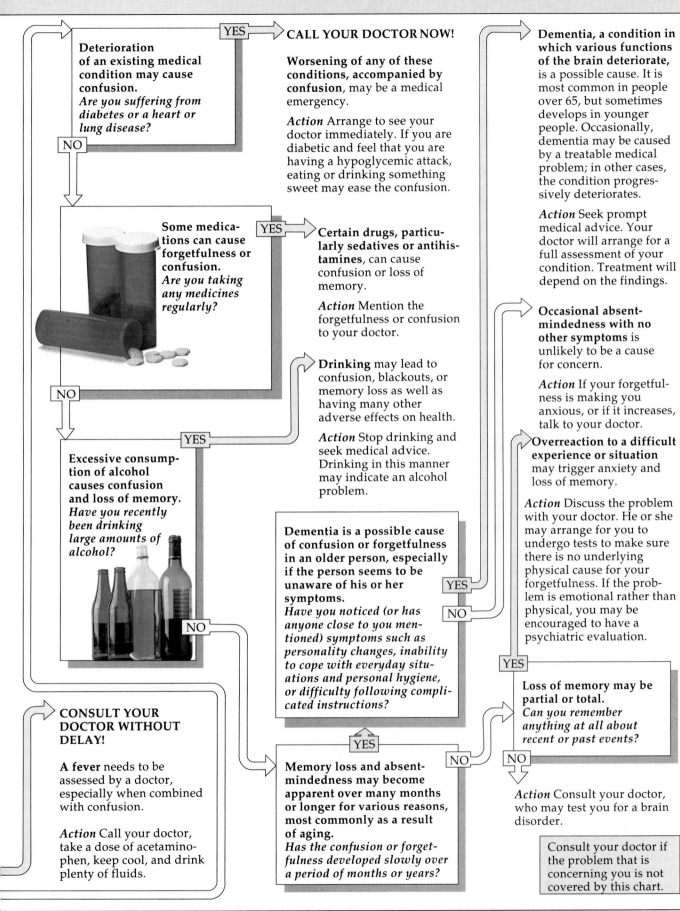

Deterioration of an existing medical condition may cause confusion. *Are you suffering from diabetes or a heart or lung disease?*

YES → **CALL YOUR DOCTOR NOW!**

Worsening of any of these conditions, accompanied by confusion, may be a medical emergency.

Action Arrange to see your doctor immediately. If you are diabetic and feel that you are having a hypoglycemic attack, eating or drinking something sweet may ease the confusion.

NO

Some medications can cause forgetfulness or confusion. *Are you taking any medicines regularly?*

YES → **Certain drugs, particularly sedatives or antihistamines,** can cause confusion or loss of memory.

Action Mention the forgetfulness or confusion to your doctor.

NO

Drinking may lead to confusion, blackouts, or memory loss as well as having many other adverse effects on health.

Action Stop drinking and seek medical advice. Drinking in this manner may indicate an alcohol problem.

YES

Excessive consumption of alcohol causes confusion and loss of memory. *Have you recently been drinking large amounts of alcohol?*

NO

Dementia is a possible cause of confusion or forgetfulness in an older person, especially if the person seems to be unaware of his or her symptoms. *Have you noticed (or has anyone close to you mentioned) symptoms such as personality changes, inability to cope with everyday situations and personal hygiene, or difficulty following complicated instructions?*

YES

NO

Dementia, a condition in which various functions of the brain deteriorate, is a possible cause. It is most common in people over 65, but sometimes develops in younger people. Occasionally, dementia may be caused by a treatable medical problem; in other cases, the condition progressively deteriorates.

Action Seek prompt medical advice. Your doctor will arrange for a full assessment of your condition. Treatment will depend on the findings.

Occasional absent-mindedness with no other symptoms is unlikely to be a cause for concern.

Action If your forgetfulness is making you anxious, or if it increases, talk to your doctor.

Overreaction to a difficult experience or situation may trigger anxiety and loss of memory.

Action Discuss the problem with your doctor. He or she may arrange for you to undergo tests to make sure there is no underlying physical cause for your forgetfulness. If the problem is emotional rather than physical, you may be encouraged to have a psychiatric evaluation.

YES

Loss of memory may be partial or total. *Can you remember anything at all about recent or past events?*

NO

CONSULT YOUR DOCTOR WITHOUT DELAY!

A fever needs to be assessed by a doctor, especially when combined with confusion.

Action Call your doctor, take a dose of acetaminophen, keep cool, and drink plenty of fluids.

YES

Memory loss and absent-mindedness may become apparent over many months or longer for various reasons, most commonly as a result of aging. *Has the confusion or forgetfulness developed slowly over a period of months or years?*

NO

Action Consult your doctor, who may test you for a brain disorder.

Consult your doctor if the problem that is concerning you is not covered by this chart.

DEMENTIA

Dementia is an overall impairment of the intellect, memory, and personality. About 2 percent of people between the ages of 65 and 75 suffer from dementia, and this figure rises to 15 percent for those over the age of 80.

What causes dementia?

Dementia is the result of specific disease processes. Dementia is usually caused by Alzheimer's disease (in which specific structural and chemical changes take place in the brain), by strokes (known as multi-infarct dementia), or by a combination of factors (mixed dementia).

It is also important to diagnose other conditions in an older person that could be confused with dementia. Strange behavior and apparent impairment of mental function may be the result of depression, social isolation, loss of hearing or sight, or even a brain tumor.

What are the signs?

The main signs of dementia are reduced learning ability, loss of initiative, aimlessness, loss of capacity for abstract thought, loss of concentration, loss of

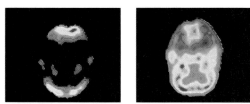

Dementia
These images, produced by positron emission tomography, show the difference in metabolic activity between a normal brain (right) and the brain of a person with dementia.

self-esteem, inattention to personal cleanliness, personality deterioration, and progressive impairment of memory, initially for recent events but later affecting long-term memory as well. The person's behavior may become increasingly uninhibited, noisy, antisocial, aggressive, or even suspicious and distrusting. He or she may become restless and wander. The person is often confused and disoriented and becomes incontinent and increasingly unable to care for himself or herself. These developments can become a great psychological and physical burden on the care giver – often a spouse.

Seeking advice

If you suspect that dementia may be developing in someone you know, seek advice from your doctor. Depending on the cause and degree of advancement of the disease, treatment may be possible. You may also get practical help from visiting nurses or from day care centers established to help ease the strain of caring for a person with dementia. Some individuals who have dementia must be placed in a nursing home.

REVERSIBLE CAUSES OF DEMENTIA

Dementia may result from:

◆ Ingesting alcohol or some medications or poisons
◆ Head injury
◆ Vitamin deficiencies, malnutrition, or dehydration
◆ Underactive thyroid gland
◆ Diabetes
◆ Oxygen deprivation to the brain (which occurs with chronic pulmonary disease or heart failure)
◆ Epilepsy
◆ Certain infections
◆ Kidney failure

MENTAL STATUS QUESTIONNAIRE

Use the test below to roughly assess the mental status of an older person who has been exhibiting unusual behavior. Give one point for each correct answer. Nineteen points is good. Less than 15 points is poor; medical advice should be sought.

1. What is your name?
2. What is your address?
3. What is the time (to the nearest hour)?
4. What day of the week is it?
5. What is the date (correct day of the month)?
6. What year is it?
7. Where are you now? What type of place is it (for example, a hospital)? Tell the person if he or she does not know and ask again at the end of the test.
8. Ask the person to remember an address. Ask the person to repeat it to ensure that he or she has heard correctly. Ask again at the end of the test.
9. Ask the person to identify two persons – for example, a neighbor, spouse, son, or daughter or a famous person in a magazine.
10. What is your date of birth (day and month)?
11. What is the city or town of your birth?
12. What school did you attend?
13. Name one of your former occupations.
14. Name your next of kin.
15. What year did World War I end?
16. What year did World War II end?
17. Who is the current president?
18. Name the months of the year backward.
19. Count from 1 to 20.
20. Count backward from 20 to 1.

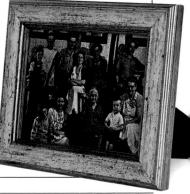

MEDICATION AND THE OLDER PERSON

As you age you become less able to metabolize drugs and excrete them from your body. Your total body mass is reduced and it is possible that you could have an adverse reaction to a drug if you take the normal adult dose. Doctors will often prescribe smaller or less frequent doses of medications for older people.

In addition, diseases of the kidney, liver, or intestine can impair the body's ability to handle some medications. For example, tetracycline is excreted by the kidneys; if the kidneys are diseased, toxic levels of tetracycline can accumulate and further kidney damage may result.

The chance of an adverse reaction to a medication increases with age. Report any unusual or unpleasant side effects to your doctor immediately.

Compliance

It is estimated that as many as two out of five people do not take their prescription drugs as directed. As you grow older, your compliance with your doctor's instructions about the dosage and timing of your medications is especially important. To make compliance easier, certain medications may be prescribed to be taken once or twice daily rather than 3 or 4 times a day. When you get a new prescription, always make sure you tell your doctor about any other medications you are taking, so that you can avoid dangerous interactions.

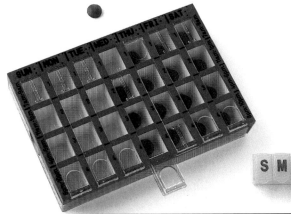

Memory aids
Special packaging, such as calendar and blister packs, is available to help older people remember when to take their medication. Compartmentalized pillboxes are also good memory aids.

SAVING MEDICATIONS

Older people may store prescription drugs for many years, forgetting to dispose of them or not wanting to waste them. In such cases, they could be taking drugs that (because they are out of date or have been stored improperly) are ineffective or even dangerous. Encourage your older relatives to dispose of unused medications after completing a course of treatment.

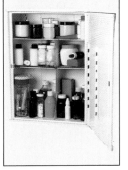

ASK YOUR DOCTOR
SPECIAL HEALTH PROBLEMS

Q **Twice recently I got up to urinate at night and almost passed out while standing at the toilet. Is there something wrong with my heart? I'm 70.**

A This sounds like micturition (urination) syncope, which affects elderly men. While you stand and your bladder empties, your blood pressure falls, which may cause fainting. Check with your doctor. It is advisable for you to sit down while urinating.

Q **My mother just turned 75 and says she has not seen a doctor for 25 years. Is there any reason for her to see a doctor now?**

A Your mother may benefit in several ways from establishing a relationship with a doctor now. The doctor can examine her carefully for "hidden" diseases such as hypertension or cancer and can give her shots for influenza and pneumonia. Your mother will also be able to get to know the doctor and develop trust in him or her. If a medical problem arises in the future, the doctor will have her records, and your mother will already have a doctor she is comfortable with.

Q **I am 75 and healthy, except for a mild case of arthritis. What is the best form of exercise for me?**

A Swimming, preferably in a heated pool, may be an ideal exercise for you because it strengthens the heart, lungs, and muscles and improves circulation, without putting any strain on your joints. Walking regularly is also an excellent all-around exercise.

APPENDIX

The material included on these four pages is designed to help you carry out some of the suggestions that were made in earlier sections of the book. The charts may be photocopied so that you will be able to use them as many times as you need. Cross-references given at the beginning of the charts refer you to relevant pages where you can find more information on each topic.

MOLE MAP

See SKIN SELF-EXAMINATION on **page 54**.

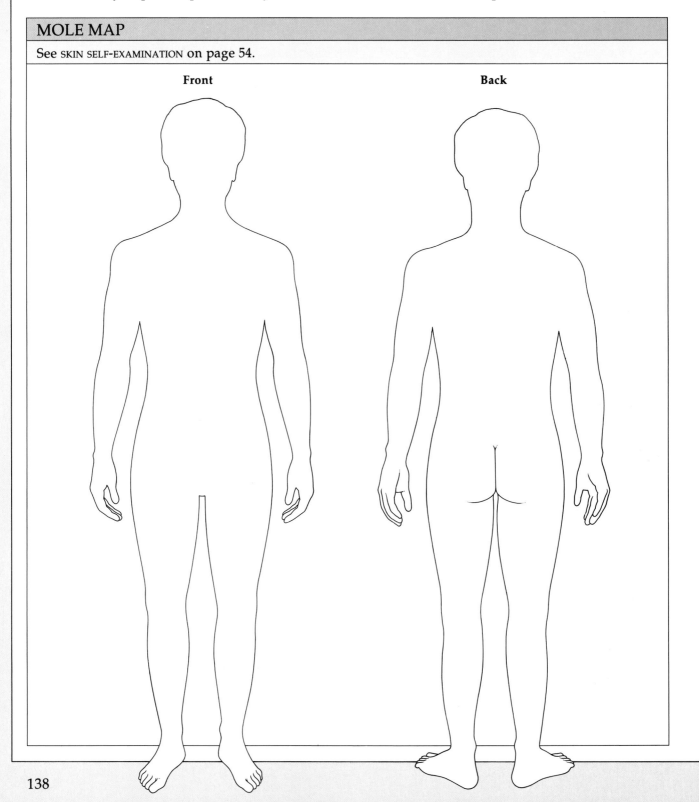

Front

Back

WEIGHT/HEIGHT CHARTS

See RISKS OF EXCESS WEIGHT on page 24.

HEIGHT (without shoes)	SMALL FRAME		MEDIUM FRAME		LARGE FRAME	
	Men	Women	Men	Women		
6'3"	157 - 168		165 - 183		175 - 197	
6'2"	153 - 164		160 - 178		171 - 192	
6'1"	149 - 160		155 - 173		166 - 187	
6'0"	145 - 155		151 - 168		161 - 182	
5'11"	141 - 151		147 - 163		157 - 177	
5'10"	137 - 147	134 - 144	143 - 158	140 - 155	152 - 172	149 - 169
5'9"	133 - 143	130 - 140	139 - 153	136 - 151	148 - 167	145 - 164
5'8"	129 - 138	126 - 136	135 - 149	132 - 147	144 - 163	141 - 159
5'7"	125 - 134	122 - 131	131 - 145	128 - 143	140 - 159	137 - 154
5'6"	121 - 130	118 - 127	127 - 140	124 - 139	135 - 154	133 - 150
5'5"	117 - 126	114 - 123	123 - 136	120 - 135	131 - 149	129 - 146
5'4"	114 - 122	110 - 119	120 - 132	116 - 131	128 - 145	125 - 142
5'3"	111 - 119	107 - 115	117 - 129	112 - 126	125 - 141	121 - 138
5'2"	108 - 116	104 - 112	114 - 126	109 - 122	122 - 137	117 - 134
5'1"	105 - 113	101 - 109	111 - 122	106 - 118	119 - 134	114 - 130
5'0"		98 - 106		103 - 115		111 - 127
4'11"		95 - 103		100 - 112		108 - 124
4'10"		92 - 100		97 - 109		105 - 121
4'9"		90 - 97		94 - 106		102 - 118
4'8"		88 - 94		92 - 103		100 - 115

PERSONAL HEALTH RECORD

CHECKUPS See the recommendations on page 17.	DATE	RESULT
Eye examination		
Dental checkup		
Cervical (Pap) smear		
Blood pressure		
Blood cholesterol		
Mammography		
Examination of rectum and colon		
Complete physical examination		

MAJOR ILLNESSES/SURGERY	DATE	TREATMENT/OUTCOME

MEDICATIONS	DATE STARTED	DATE STOPPED	ADVERSE REACTIONS

WEEKLY ALCOHOL INTAKE

See DRINKING ALCOHOL on pages 112 to 117.

Fill in the chart below for at least 1 week. Count the following as one drink – a 3.5-ounce glass of wine, a 1.5-ounce shot of hard liquor, and a 12-ounce glass of regular (not light) beer. Remember, however, that different types of wine or beer contain different percentages of alcohol and that home measurements often tend to be generous. Show the chart to your doctor.

DAY	TIME	PLACE AND ACTIVITY	TYPE OF DRINK	AMOUNT	DAY'S TOTAL
Mon					
Tue					
Wed					
Thur					
Fri					
Sat					
Sun					
				WEEK'S TOTAL	

DAILY SMOKING PATTERN

See SMOKING on pages 110 to 112.

If you have decided to follow the advice about quitting smoking on page 112, fill in each column in the chart below every time you light up during the day. Under AMOUNT, record how much of the cigarette/cigar/pipe you actually smoked. Try to quit smoking completely.

DATE	TIME	PLACE AND ACTIVITY	REASON(S)	AMOUNT

IMMUNIZATIONS FOR TRAVEL ABROAD

See FOREIGN TRAVEL on page 101.

IMMUNIZATION	REASONS FOR IMMUNIZATION	METHOD AND EFFECTIVENESS	DATE OF LAST IMMUNIZATION OR BOOSTER
Yellow fever	Compulsory for entry into some countries and recommended for visits to others within yellow fever zones in Africa, South America, and Central America.	Single injection gives the traveler nearly 100 percent protection for at least 10 years.	
Typhoid	Recommended for travel anywhere outside of the US, Canada, Northern Europe, Australia, and New Zealand for anyone who has not received immunization or a booster within the past 5 years.	Two injections given 28 days apart give moderate to good protection for about 5 years. After that, a booster is needed.	
Cholera	Occasionally compulsory for entry into some countries in Asia and Africa during cholera epidemics, although this may create a false sense of security, since the vaccine is only partially effective. Most authorities do not ever recommend routine vaccination.	Two injections given 14 to 28 days apart give mild protection for 6 months. After that, a booster is needed.	
Poliomyelitis	Recommended for anyone who has not received childhood immunization or a booster within the past 10 years.	Childhood immunization, consisting of three doses and a booster at 4 to 6 years, is highly effective. More boosters are needed every 10 years.	
Tetanus	Recommended for anyone who has not received childhood immunization or a booster within the past 10 years.	Childhood immunization, consisting of three doses with a booster at 4 to 6 years, is highly effective. More boosters are needed every 10 years.	
Immune serum globulin	Recommended when traveling where hygiene and sanitary standards are low, to protect against viral hepatitis type A.	Moderate protection is provided for up to 3 months.	

NOTES

1. MALARIA PREVENTION Medication for the prevention of malaria is required for travel to many parts of tropical and subtropical regions. Ask your doctor for advice.

2. OTHER PRECAUTIONS To help protect yourself against diseases such as typhoid, viral hepatitis type A, and diarrheal illnesses in areas where standards of hygiene are low, take adequate precautions with food and drink. Drink only bottled drinks or boiled water, and avoid eating salads, unpeeled fruit, shellfish, undercooked meat, or dairy products such as ice cream.

See TEST YOUR SHORT-TERM MEMORY on page 77.

INDEX

Page numbers in *italics* refer to illustrations and captions.

Photograph sources:
Adams Picture Library **13** (bottom right)
Aid-Call **131**
Alcoholics Anonymous, World Services, Inc. **117**
The American Cancer Society **16**
Art Directors Photo Library **13** (bottom left)
Aspect Picture Library Ltd **101** (top left)
St. Bartholomew's Hospital **38** (bottom far right); **43** (bottom center)
Bridgeman Art Library **78** (inset)
British Nuclear Fuels (Sellafield) **95** (bottom left)
John Browett **121** (top); **121** (bottom)
Dr Martin Edwards **38** (bottom right)
Environmental Picture Library **98** (bottom left); **99** (bottom left)
Greg Evans Photo Library **124** (top left)
Susan Griggs Agency Ltd **83** (bottom)
The Image Bank **9**; **25**; **33 (top)**; **56** (bottom); **71** (bottom left, bottom right, bottom right center, top left); **91** (center left, bottom left); **95** (top); **98** (top right); **99** (bottom left); **107** (bottom); **123** (bottom); **125** (bottom); **127** (top); **131** (top right)
National Medical Slide Bank, UK **18** (top); **40** (top right, center, bottom right); **41** (top right, center left, center middle, center right); **42** (top right inset); **43** (top

left, top center, center left, top right, center middle, bottom right); **46** (top left, top right); **47**; **52**; **115** (left); **129**
Pictor International **21**; **69**; **85**; **119**; **125** (top); **126**
Picture point Ltd **122**
Planet Earth Pictures **99** (background)
Rex Features **113**
Sealand Aerial Photography **23** (center)
Science Photo Library **19** (right); **39** (bottom left); **41**(bottom left); **42** (top left); **43** (center right); **46** (bottom left, center left, center right); **54** (bottom right); **76**; **94** (left); **94** (right); **129**; **136**
Spectrum Colour Library **99** (top right)
Tony Stone Worldwide **34** (top); **71** (bottom left center); **71** (top right); **95** (bottom right)
Elizabeth Whiting & Associates **97** (top)
Dr Ian Williams **42** (top right); **54** (bottom center)
Dr Robert Youngson **35** (bottom left); **35** (bottom right)
Dr J. Zakrzewska **38** (bottom far left); **38** (bottom left); **38** (bottom center)
Zefa **54** (bottom left); **58**; **87**; **91** (top left); **99** (center left); **99** (center right); **101** (top right)

Front cover photograph: © 1988 Michael Keller / The Stock Market

Commissioned photography:
Susanna Price
Steve Bartholomew

Illustrators:
Russell Barnet
Karen Cochrane
David Fathers
Tony Graham
Andrew Green
John Woodcock

Peter Bull
Marks Illustration and Design
Gilly Newman

Airbrushing:
Janos Marffy
Trevor Hill
Roy Flooks

Index:
Susan Bosanko

The photograph on page 29 was taken on the premises of the Rock Garden Cafe, Covent Garden, London.

The 1-Mile Walking Test on pages 23-24 was developed by and provided courtesy of The Institute For Aerobics Research, Dallas, Texas.